The Comprehensive Vegetarian Lunch & Soup Cookbook

Easy Vegetarian Lunch And Soup Dishes For Everyone

Adam Denton

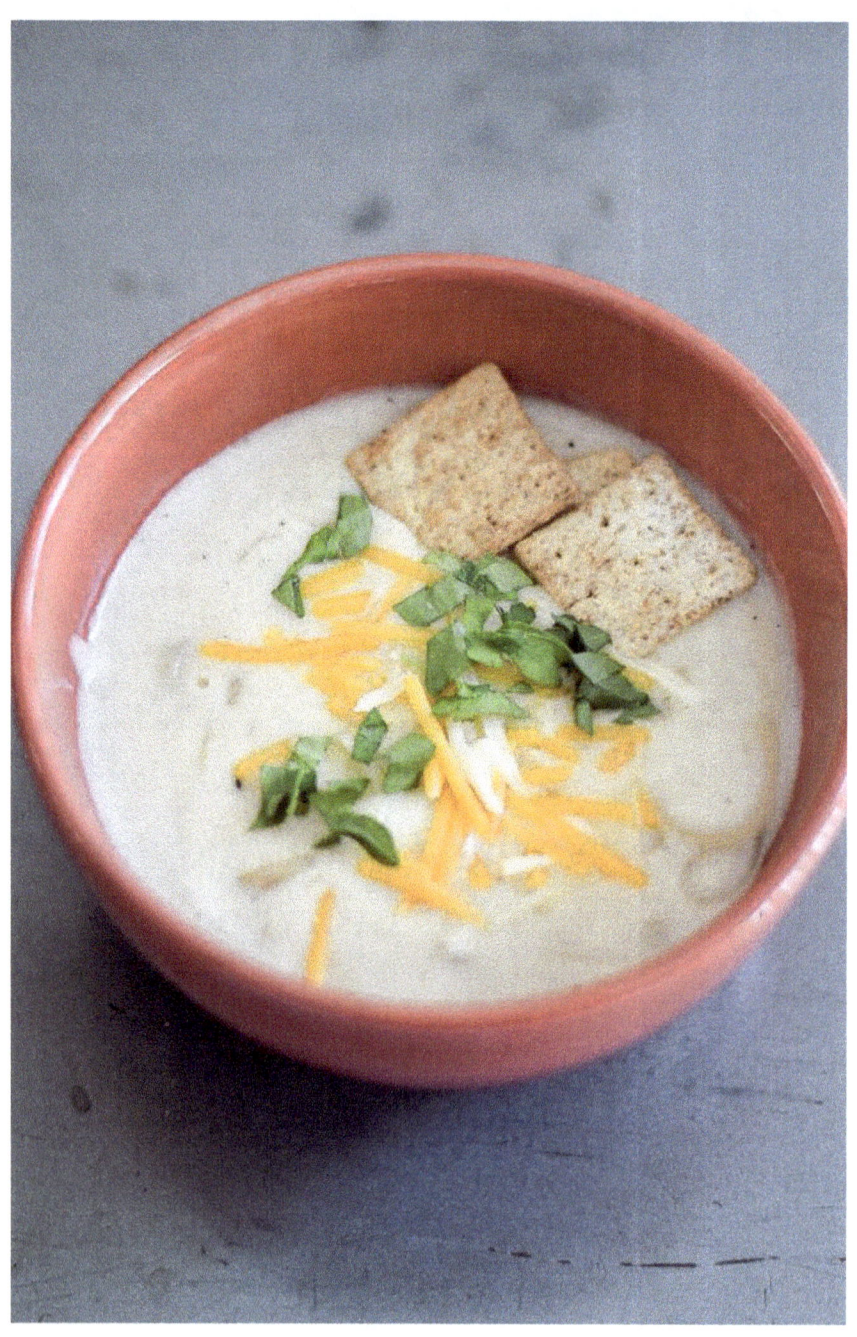

© Copyright 2020 - All rights reserved.

The content contained within this book may not be reproduced, duplicated or transmitted without direct written permission from the author or the publisher.

Under no circumstances will any blame or legal responsibility be held against the publisher, or author, for any damages, reparation, or monetary loss due to the information contained within this book. Either directly or indirectly.

Legal Notice:

This book is copyright protected. This book is only for personal use. You cannot amend, distribute, sell, use, quote or paraphrase any part, or the content within this book, without the consent of the author or publisher.

Disclaimer Notice:

Please note the information contained within this document is for educational and entertainment purposes only. All effort has been executed to present accurate, up to date, and reliable, complete information. No warranties of any kind are declared or implied. Readers acknowledge that the author is not engaging in the rendering of legal, financial, medical or professional advice. The content within this book has been derived from various sources. Please consult a licensed professional before attempting any techniques outlined in this book.

By reading this document, the reader agrees that under no circumstances is the author responsible for any losses, direct or indirect, which are incurred as a result of the use of information contained within this document, including, but not limited to, — errors, omissions, or inaccuracies.

Table of contents

Creamy Squash and Poblano Pepper Soup 7

Summer Squash Fenugreek Soup 10

Summer Squash Curry Soup 12

Butternut Squash and Mung Bean Soup 14

Turnip and Tarragon Soup 16

Thai Carrot Soup 18

Carrot and Kalamata Olive Soup 20

Spicy Turnip and Onion Soup 22

Vidalia Onion Soup 24

Tomato and Lentil Soup 26

Asian Spinach and Soybean Soup 28

Lentils and Sun-dried Tomato Soup 30

Spicy Jalapeno Soy Bean Soup 32

Smoky Summer Squash and Carrot Soup 34

Chinese Butternut Squash Soup 36

Winter Squash Carrot and Cayenne Pepper Soup 38

Winter Squash and Carrots Soup 40

Lima Bean Soup 42

Sesame and Soy Bean Soup 44

Jalapeno Tortilla Soup 46

Vegan Chorizo and White Bean Tortilla Soup 48

Parsnip and Turnip Soup 50

Jalapeno Turnip and Carrot Soup 52

Ancho Chili Carrot and Turnip Soup 53

Hungarian Winter Squash and Carrot Soup 55

Poblano Chili and Summer Squash Soup 57

Creamy Potato Soup Poblano Soup 60

Borlotti Bean and Squash Soup 63

Spicy Summer Squash and Lentil Soup 65

Chinese Turnip Soup 67

Garnish with cilantro Spicy and Tangy Parsnip Soup 69

Italian Vidalia Onion Soup 71

French Parsnip and Tarragon Soup 73

Pesto Carrot and Turnip Soup 75

Red Onion Turnip Soup 77

Roasted Sweet Potatoes and Green Bean Soup 78

Spicy Tomato and Sweet Potato Soup 81

Baked Smoky Broccoli and Garlic 84

Asian Roasted Broccoli and Choy Sum 86

Roasted Cauliflower and Lima Beans 87

Roasted Brussel Sprouts and Choy Sum 89

Thai Roasted Spicy Black Beans and Choy Sum 90

Simple Roasted Broccoli and Cauliflower 92

Roasted Spinach and Mustard Greens Extra 94

Roasted Napa Cabbage and Turnips Extra 96

Simple Roasted Kale Artichoke Heart and Choy Sum Extra 97

Chinese Roasted Button Mushrooms and Butternut Squash 98

Roasted Kale and Bok Choy Extra 100

Roasted Lima Beans and Summer Squash.. 102

Roasted Soy Beans and Winter Squash 105

Creamy Squash and Poblano Pepper Soup

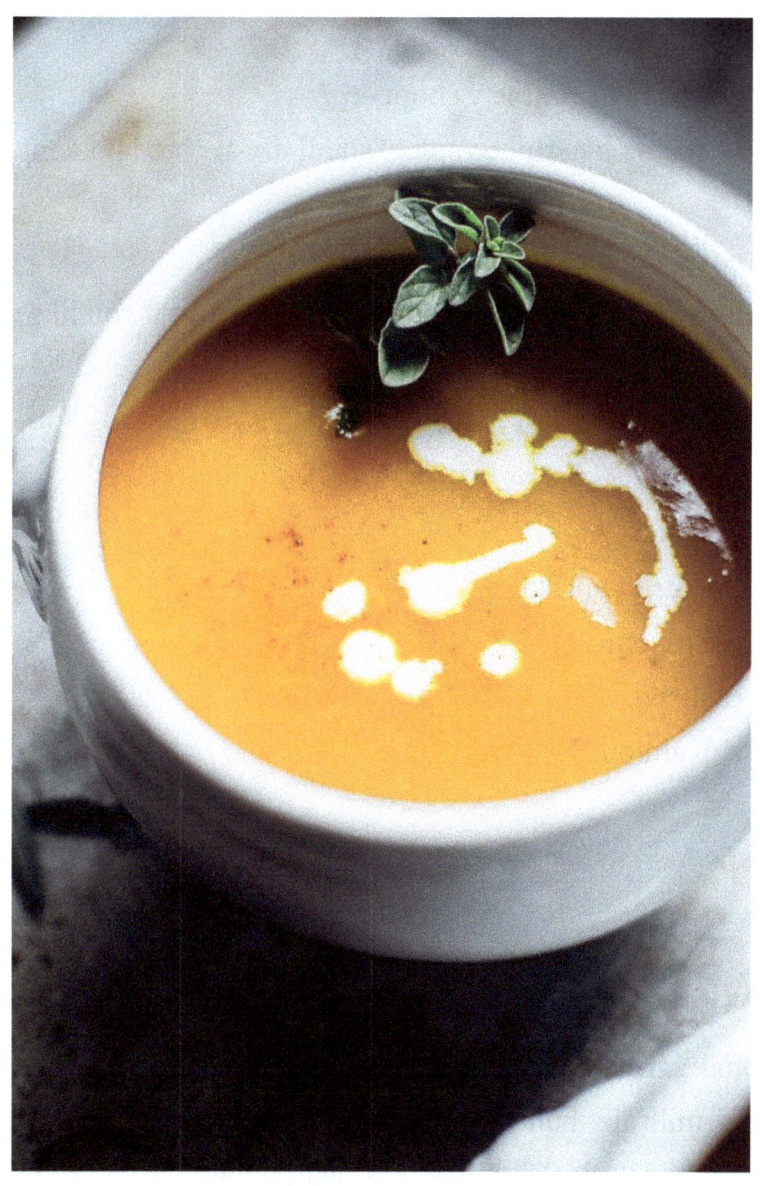

Ingredients:

4 tablespoons organic unsalted butter

1 small red onion, coarsely chopped

1 large leek, white part only, sliced

1 red bell pepper, coarsely chopped

1 (or two if you like things spicy) small dry-roasted poblano chili, sliced

4 cloves garlic, diced

1 small summer squash, cubed (you can use two if you like your soup thick)

4 cups vegetable broth

2 tsp. cumin

1 tsp. oregano

1 tsp. Spanish paprika

1 dash of cayenne pepper

1 cup cashews

1-1/4 cup almond milk

Sea Salt

Black pepper, to taste+

Directions:

Optional garnish: Sliced jalapeno pepper Soak the cashews in almond milk for half an hour. Melt non-dairy butter in a pan. Cook the onion, leek, chilies, red bell pepper, garlic, and potato over low heat until the onion is translucent. Add the broth , cumin, oregano, paprika and cayenne pepper into the pan. Simmer until the potatoes are fork tender, about 25 min. Remove from the heat. Pour into a blender and blend until smooth. Clean the blender. Blend cashews with the milk until smooth Stir this into the soup. Heat on medium for a few minutes. Garnish with slices of jalapeno chili.

Summer Squash Fenugreek Soup

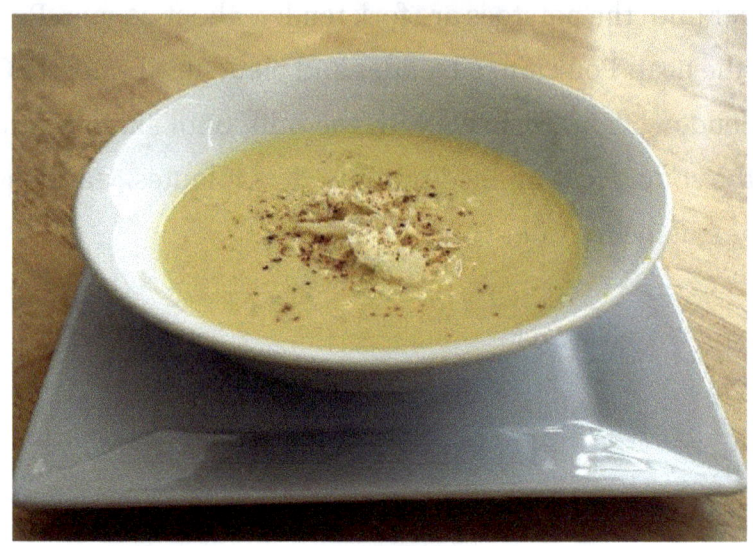

Ingredients

1 tablespoon extra virgin olive oil

1 small red onion, chopped

1 tablespoon minced fresh ginger root

5 cloves garlic, chopped

1 pinch fenugreek seeds

1 cup dry red lentils

1 cup summer squash - peeled, seeded, and cubed

1/3 cup finely chopped fresh cilantro

2 cups water

2 tablespoons honey

1/8 teaspoon ground cinnamon

1 pinch ground nutmeg

salt and pepper to taste

Directions:

Heat the pot over medium heat Sauté the onion, ginger, garlic, and fenugreek until onion is tender. Add the lentils, squash, and cilantro into the pot. Add the water, coconut milk, and tomato paste. Add the curry powder, cayenne pepper, nutmeg, salt, and pepper. Boil, reduce the heat to low, and simmer until lentils and squash are tender for 25 min.

Summer Squash Curry Soup

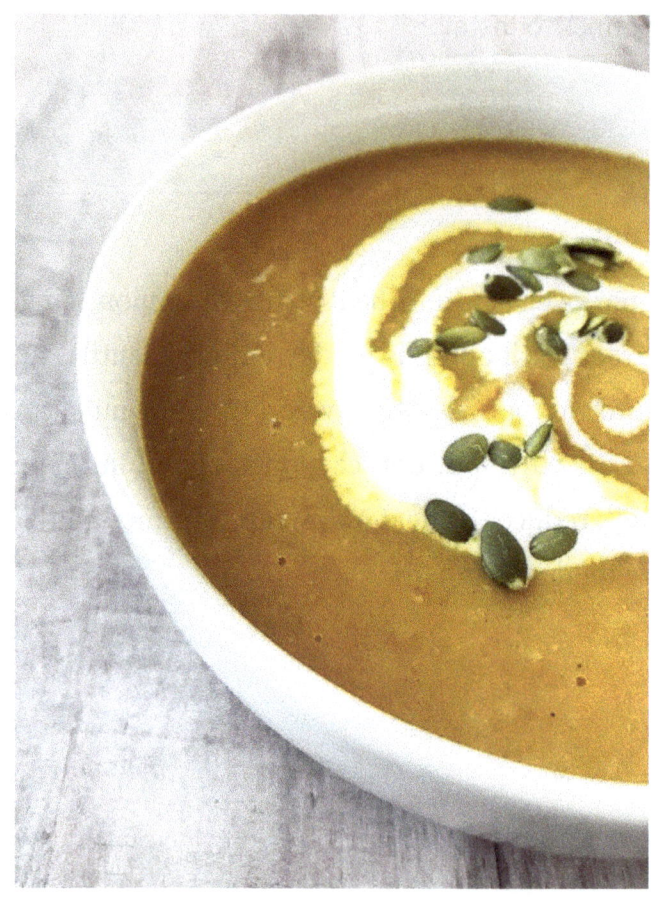

Ingredients

1 tablespoon extra virgin olive oil

1 small red onion, chopped

1 tablespoon minced fresh ginger root

4 cloves garlic, chopped

1 cup dry red lentils

1 cup summer squash - peeled, seeded, and cubed

1/3 cup finely chopped fresh coriander

2 cups water

1/2 (14 ounce) can coconut milk

½ teaspoon ground cumin

1 teaspoon red curry powder

1/2 tsp. garam masala

1 pinch ground turmeric

salt and pepper to taste

Directions:

Heat the pot over medium heat Sauté the onion, ginger, and garlic until onion is tender. Add the lentils, squash, and coriander into the pot. Add the water & coconut milk Add the curry powder, cumin, garam masala, turmeric, salt, and pepper. Boil, reduce the heat to low, and simmer until lentils and squash are tender for 25 min.

Butternut Squash and Mung Bean Soup

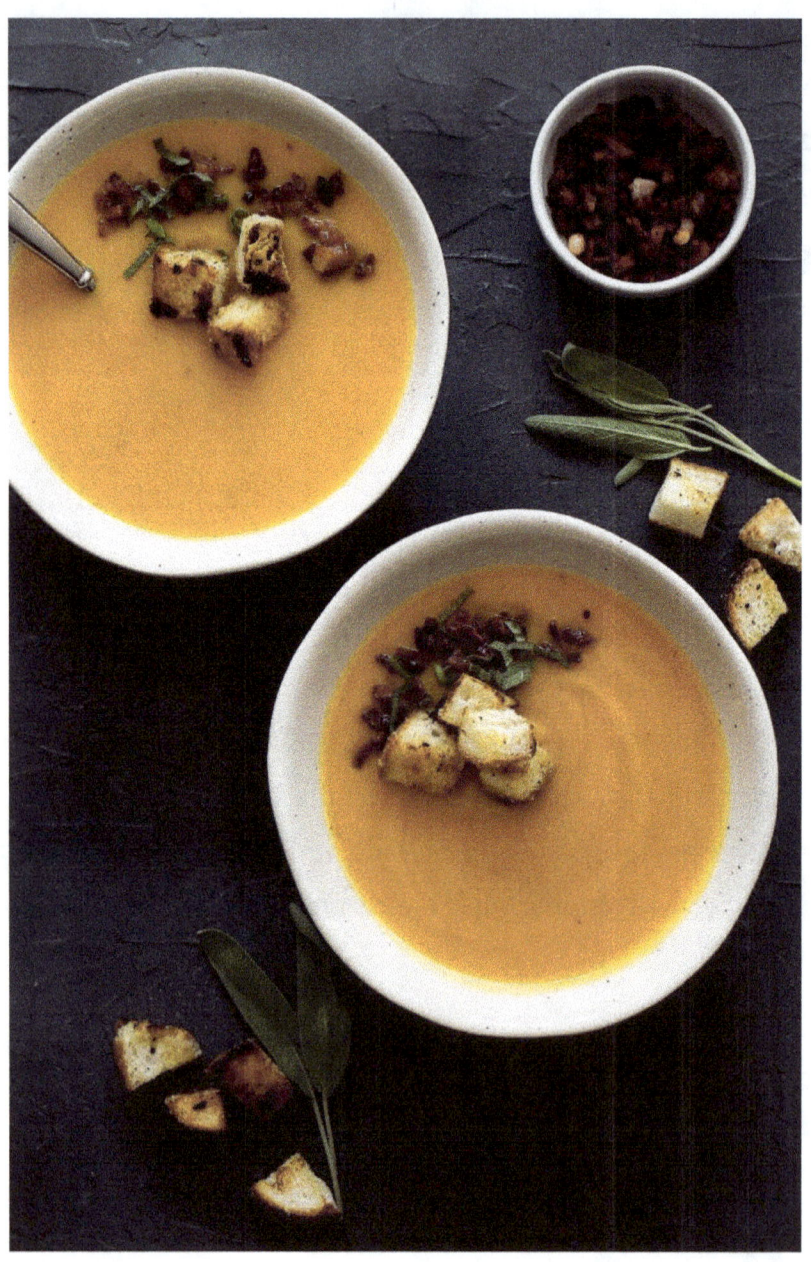

Ingredients

3 tablespoons extra virgin olive oil

1 small red onion, chopped

1 tablespoon minced fresh ginger root

4 cloves garlic, chopped

1 pinch fenugreek seeds

1 cup dry mung beans

1 cup butternut squash - peeled, seeded, and cubed

1/3 cup finely chopped fresh cilantro

2 ½ cups vegetable broth

2 tablespoons tomato paste

1 teaspoon Italian seasoning

¼ tsp. cayenne pepper

1 pinch thyme

salt and pepper to taste

Directions:

Heat the pot over medium heat Sauté the red onion, ginger, garlic, and fenugreek until onion is tender. Add the beans, squash, and cilantro into the pot. Add the broth and tomato paste. Add the Italian seasoning, cayenne pepper, thyme, salt, and pepper. Boil, reduce the heat to low, and simmer until lentils and squash are tender for 25 min.

Turnip and Tarragon Soup

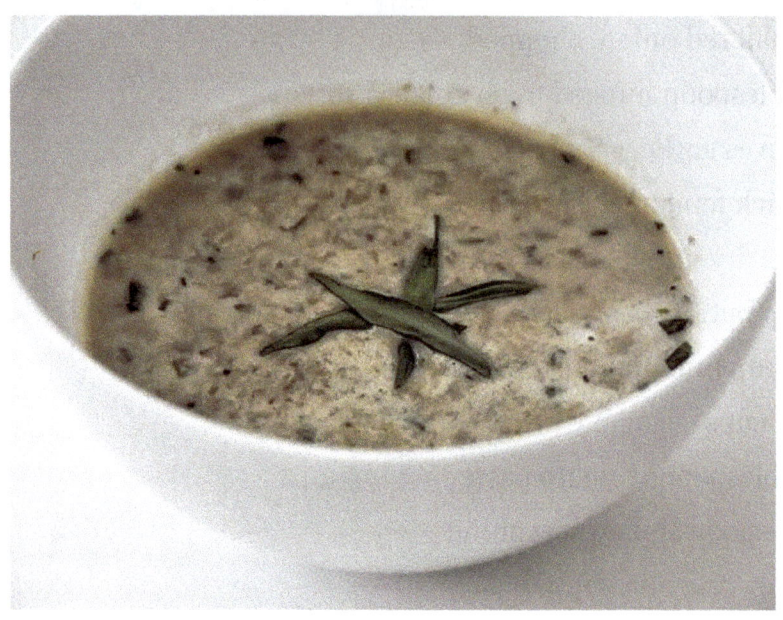

Ingredients

3 tablespoons extra virgin olive oil

1 small red onion, minced

1 small turnip, peeled and thinly sliced

1 celery rib, thinly sliced

1/2 teaspoon dried tarragon

2 cups vegetable broth

2 tbsp. white wine vinegar

Directions:

Heat oil over medium-high heat. Sauté onions until tender for about 5 minutes. Add turnip, celery, and tarragon, and cook for another 5 minutes, or until carrots become tender. Add vegetable broth and wine vinegar. Boil and reduce to a simmer, and cook for 15 minutes longer.

Thai Carrot Soup

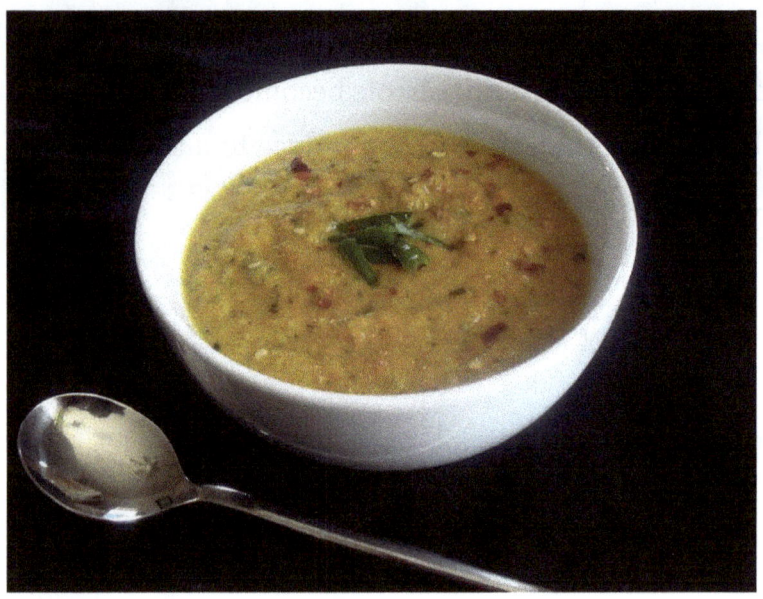

Ingredients

3 tablespoons sesame seed oil

1 small red onion, minced

1 small carrot, peeled and thinly sliced

1 celery rib, thinly sliced

1/2 teaspoon Thai bird chilies

2 cups vegetable broth

2 tbsp. sherry vinegar

Directions:

Heat sesame oil over medium-high heat. Sauté onions until tender for about 5 minutes. Add carrots, celery, and Thai bird chilies, and cook for another 5 minutes, or until carrots become tender. Add vegetable broth and sherry vinegar. Boil and reduce to a simmer, and cook for 15 minutes longer.

Carrot and Kalamata Olive Soup

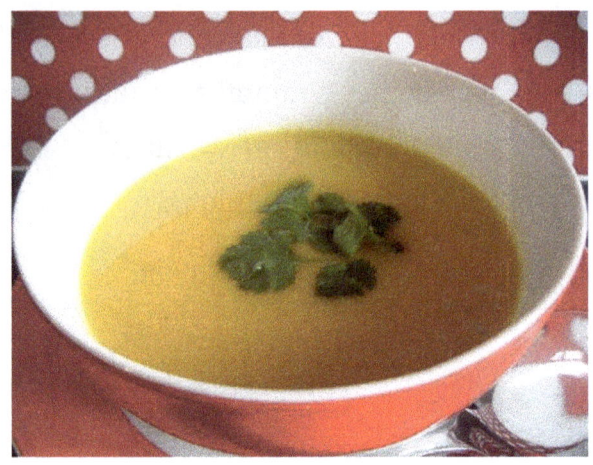

Ingredients

3 tablespoons melted salted butter

1 small red onion, minced

1 small carrot, peeled and thinly sliced

1 celery rib, thinly sliced

8 pcs. kalamata olives

2 tsp. lemon juice

9 cloves garlic, minced

1/2 teaspoon cumin

2 cups vegetable broth

2 tbsp. white wine vinegar

Directions:

Heat butter over medium-high heat. Sauté onions and garlic until tender for about 5 minutes. Add carrots, celery, and tarragon, cumin and cook for another 5 minutes, or until carrots become tender. Add vegetable broth, kalamata olives, capers and lemon juice and wine vinegar. Boil and reduce to a simmer, and cook for 15 minutes longer.

Spicy Turnip and Onion Soup

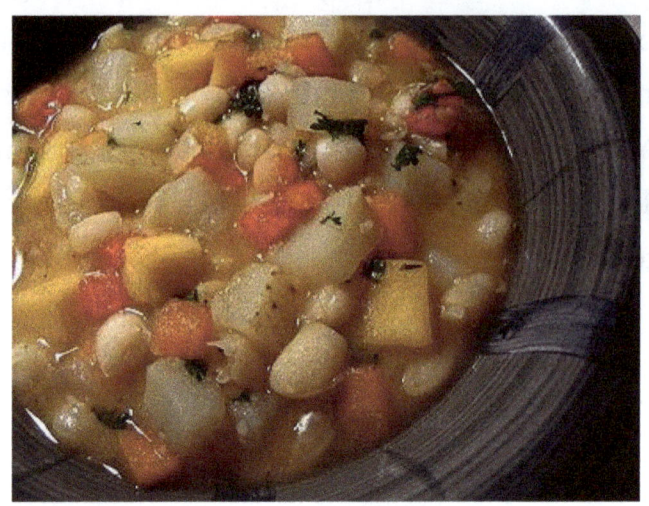

Ingredients

3 tablespoons extra virgin olive oil

1 large red onion, minced

1 small turnip, peeled and thinly sliced

1 ancho chili , thinly sliced

1/2 teaspoon cumin

½ tsp. cayenne pepper

1 cup vegetable broth

1 cup vegetable stock

2 tbsp. white wine vinegar

Directions:

Heat oil over medium-high heat. Sauté onions until tender for about 5 minutes. Add turnip, ancho chili, cumin and cayenne pepper, and cook for another 5 minutes, or until turnip become tender. Add vegetable broth, vegetable stock and wine vinegar. Boil and reduce to a simmer, and cook for 15 minutes longer.

Vidalia Onion Soup

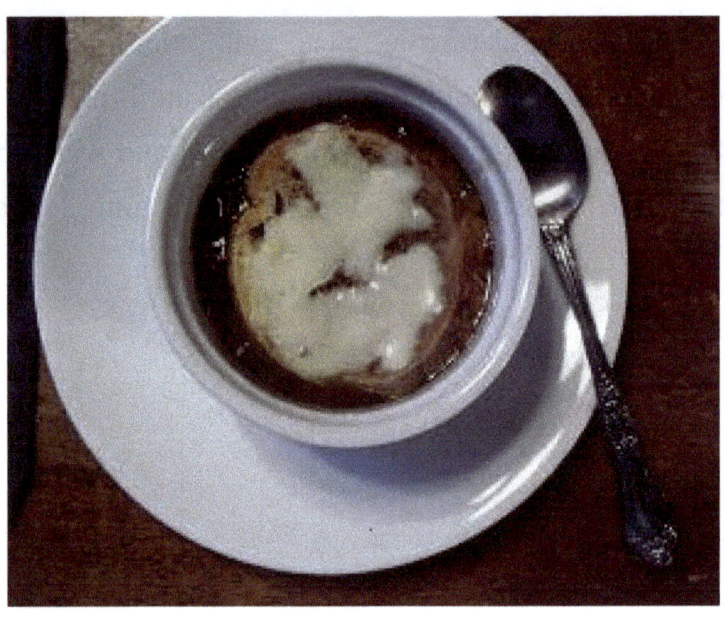

Ingredients

3 tablespoons extra virgin olive oil

1 Vidalia onion, minced

1 small carrot, peeled and thinly sliced

1 celery rib, thinly sliced

1/2 teaspoon dried tarragon

2 cups vegetable broth

2 tbsp. white wine vinegar

Directions:

Heat oil over medium-high heat. Sauté onions until tender for about 5 minutes. Add carrots, celery, and tarragon, and cook for another 5 minutes, or until carrots become tender. Add vegetable broth and wine vinegar. Boil and reduce to a simmer, and cook for 15 minutes longer.

Tomato and Lentil Soup

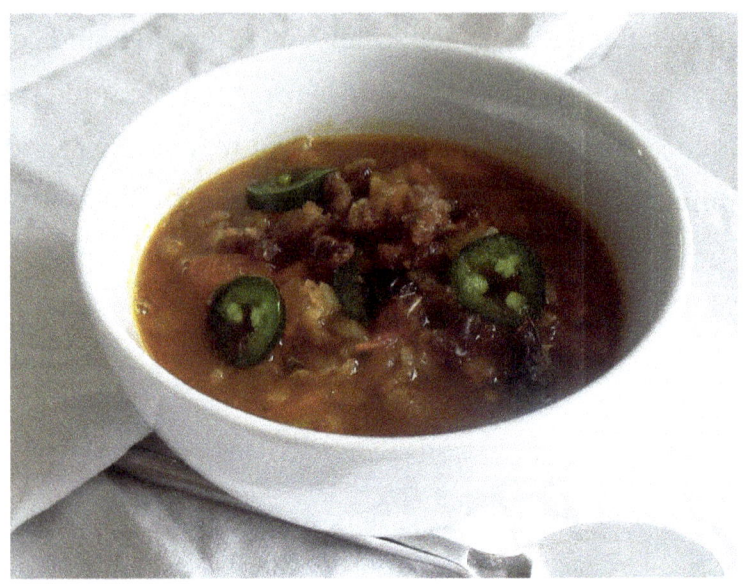

Ingredients

1 pound lentils, sorted and rinsed

1 1/2 quarts vegetable stock

½ quart water

1 medium onion, diced

6 cloves of garlic, peeled and smashed

2 tsp sea salt

1/4 tsp pepper

2 medium potatoes, diced

1 pound frozen, sliced carrots

1 cup chopped sun-dried tomatoes*

1-2 tsp dried dill

3-4 tbsp fresh, minced parsley

Directions:

Add the lentils, veggie stock and water, onion, garlic, salt and pepper in a pot and cook over low-medium heat. Simmer for 3-4 hours. When the lentils become soft, add the potato and simmer until the potatoes become tender. Add the carrots, tomatoes and dill and cook until heated through. Add the parsley. Season with more salt and pepper.

Asian Spinach and Soybean Soup

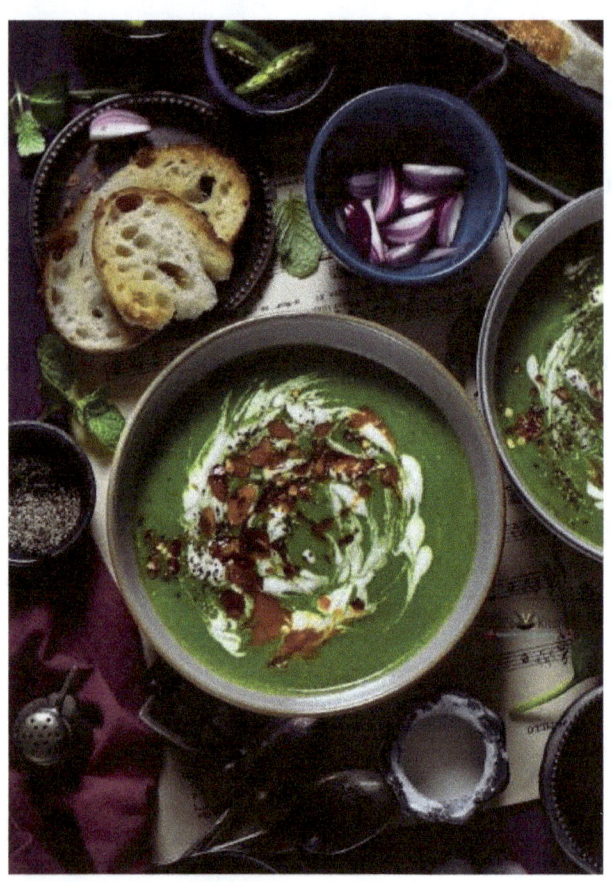

Ingredients

3/4 pound soy beans, sorted and rinsed

1 1/2 quarts vegetable stock

½ quart coconut milk

½ quart water

1 medium onion, diced

6 cloves of garlic, peeled and smashed

2 tsp sea salt

1/4 tsp pepper

1 bunch spinach, diced

1 pound frozen, sliced carrots

1-2 tsp minced ginger

3-4 tbsp fresh, minced parsley

Directions:

Add the beans, vegetable stock, coconut milk and water, onion, garlic, salt and pepper in a pot and cook over low-medium heat. Simmer for 3-4 hours. When the beans become soft, add the spinach and simmer until the potatoes become tender. Add the carrots, tomatoes and ginger and cook until heated through. Add the parsley. Season with more salt and pepper.

Lentils and Sun-dried Tomato Soup

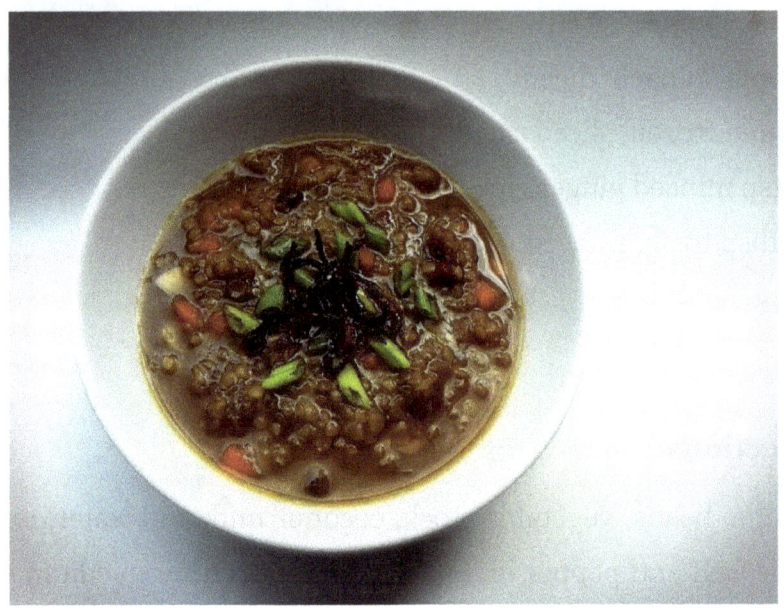

Ingredients

1 pound lentils, sorted and rinsed

1 1/2 quarts vegetable stock

½ quart water

1 medium onion, diced

6 cloves of garlic, peeled and smashed

2 tsp sea salt

1/4 tsp pepper

2 medium parsnips, diced

1 pound frozen, sliced carrots

1 cup chopped sun-dried tomatoes*

1-2 tsp ground sumac

1 tsp. thyme

1 tsp. mint

Add the lentils, veggie stock and water, onion, garlic, salt and pepper in a pot and cook over low-medium heat.

Directions:

Simmer for 3-4 hours. When the lentils become soft, add the parsnips and simmer until the parsnips become tender. Add the carrots, tomatoes, thyme and mint and cook until heated through. Season with more salt and pepper.

Spicy Jalapeno Soy Bean Soup

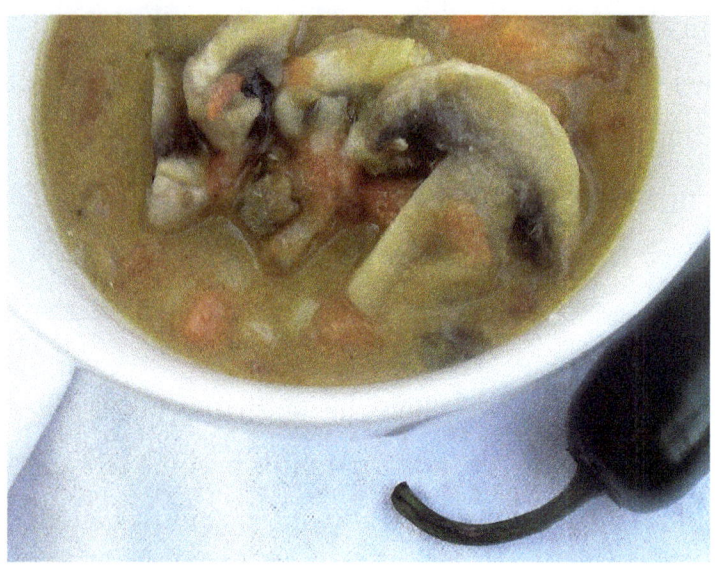

Ingredients

1 pound dry soy beans, sorted and rinsed

1 1/2 quarts vegetable stock

½ quart water

1 medium onion, diced

6 cloves of garlic, peeled and smashed

2 tsp sea salt

1/2 tsp cumin

2 ancho chilies, diced

1 pound frozen, sliced carrots

1 cup chopped sun-dried tomatoes*

1-2 tsp. dried cayenne pepper

1-2 tsp. jalapeno pepper, minced

3-4 tbsp fresh, minced parsley

Directions:

Add the beans, veggie stock and water, onion, garlic, salt and cumin in a pot and cook over low-medium heat. Simmer for 3-4 hours. When the beans become soft, add the ancho chilies and simmer until the potatoes become tender. Add the carrots, tomatoes and dill and cook until heated through. Add the cayenne pepper and jalapeno peppers. Season with more salt and pepper.

Smoky Summer Squash and Carrot Soup

Ingredients

1 medium summer squash (1 lb of peeled and cubed butternut squash)

1 medium red onion, diced

1/2 lb carrots, peeled and cut into chunks

1 Fuji apple, peeled and sliced

3 cups vegetable stock

1 cup vegetable broth

1 tsp. ground cumin

31 tsp salt

1 tsp. ground coriander

1/4 tsp dried ground sage

salt and pepper to taste

Directions:

Combine the squash, red onion, carrots, apple, broth, stock and bay leaf in slow cooker. Cook for about 6 hours on low or until veggies are soft. Take the bay leaf and discard. Transfer the Ingredients of the slow cooker to a blender Blend until smooth. Pour back into the slow cooker and season with salt, pepper, coriander, & cumin Taste and season with more salt and pepper to taste.

Chinese Butternut Squash Soup

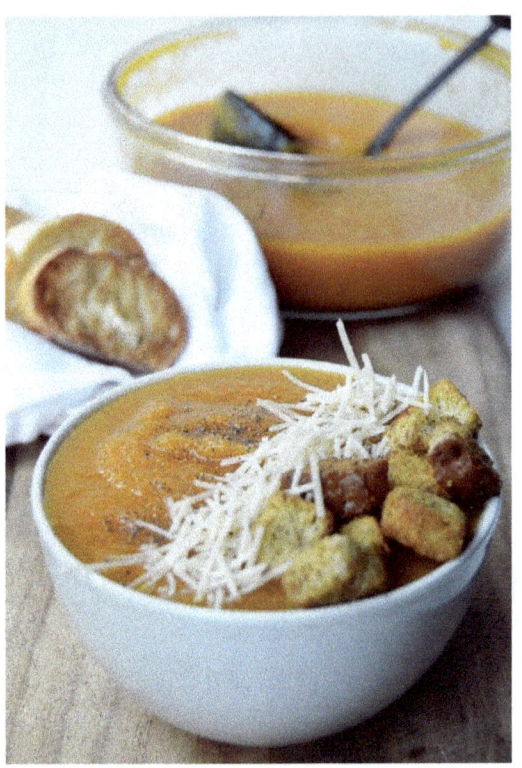

Ingredients

1 medium butternut squash (1 lb of peeled and cubed butternut squash)

1 medium red onion, diced

1/2 lb carrots, peeled and cut into chunks

3 cloves garlic, minced

3 cups vegetable stock

4 tsp. Chinese five spice powder

31 tsp salt

31 tsp pepper

1 tsp. grated ginger

1 (13.5 oz) can vegetable broth

3 tbsp. sesame seed oil

salt and pepper to taste

Directions:

Combine the squash, red onion, carrots, garlic, stock , sesame seed oil and bay leaf in slow cooker. Cook for about 6 hours on low or until veggies are soft. Take the bay leaf and discard. Transfer the Ingredients of the slow cooker to a blender Blend until smooth. Pour back into the slow cooker and season with salt, pepper & sage Add the coconut milk. Stir. Taste and season with more salt and pepper to taste.

Winter Squash Carrot and Cayenne Pepper Soup

Ingredients

1 medium winter squash

1 medium red onion, diced

1/2 lb carrots, peeled and cut into chunks

3 garlic cloves , minced

3 cups vegetable stock

31 tsp salt

31 tsp cayenne pepper

1/4 cup peanut butter

1 (13.5 oz) can coconut milk

salt and pepper to taste

Directions:

Combine the squash, red onion, carrots, peanut butter, garlic, stock and bay leaf in slow cooker. Cook for about 6 hours on low or until veggies are soft. Take the bay leaf and discard. Transfer the Ingredients of the slow cooker to a blender Blend until smooth. Pour back into the slow cooker and season with salt, pepper & sage Add the coconut milk. Stir. Taste and season with more salt and cayenne pepper to taste.

Winter Squash and Carrots Soup

Ingredients

1 medium winter squash (1 lb of peeled and cubed butternut squash)
1 medium red onion, diced
1/2 lb carrots, peeled and cut into chunks
1 Fuji apple, peeled and sliced
3 cups vegetable stock
1 fresh tarragon
31 tsp salt
31 tsp pepper
1/4 tsp herbs de Provence
salt and pepper to taste

Directions:

Combine the squash, red onion, carrots, apple, stock and fresh tarragon in slow cooker. Cook for about 6 hours on low or until veggies are soft. Take the tarragon and discard. Transfer the Ingredients of the slow cooker to a blender Blend until smooth. Pour back into the slow cooker and season with salt, pepper &

herbs de Provence Taste and season with more salt and pepper to taste.

Lima Bean Soup

Ingredients

1 teaspoon extra virgin olive oil

1/2 cup chopped red onions

4 cloves garlic, minced

2 cups vegetable broth

1 cup salsa

1 14-ounce can lima beans

1 green bell pepper, chopped

1/2 teaspoon sea salt

1 avocado, chopped

1/2 cup loosely-packed cilantro

Directions:

Optional:

1/2 cup crumbled corn tortilla chips Chop onions and garlic. Chop red bell pepper. Cook and Serve: Heat the olive oil on medium. Add the red onions and garlic to the pan and stir until softened, 3 to 5 minutes. Pour in broth, salsa, bell peppers, black beans, and salt. Boil over high heat. Reduce heat to low and simmer until heated through for about 5 minutes. Top with half of the avocado, cilantro, and tortilla chips.

Sesame and Soy Bean Soup

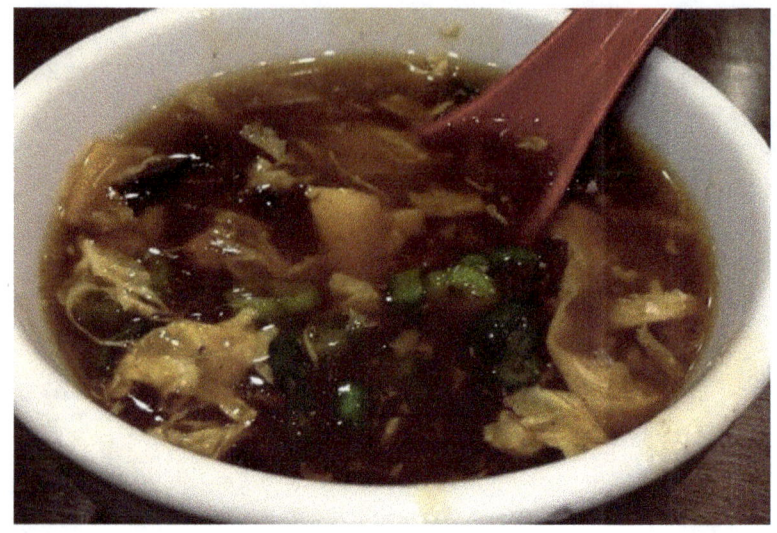

Ingredients

1 teaspoon sesame oil

1/2 cup chopped red onions

4 cloves garlic, minced

2 cups vegetable broth

1 14-ounce can soy beans

1/2 teaspoon sea salt

Directions:

Heat the sesame oil on medium. Add the red onions and garlic to the pan and stir until softened, 3 to 5 minutes. Pour in broth, black beans, and salt. Boil over high heat. Reduce heat to low and simmer until heated through for about 5 minutes.

Jalapeno Tortilla Soup

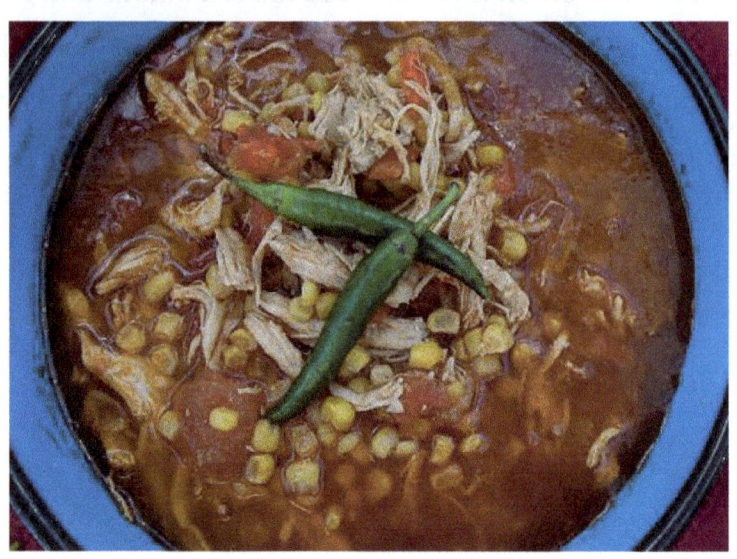

Ingredients:

1 teaspoon extra virgin olive oil

1/2 cup chopped red onions

4 cloves garlic, minced

2 cups vegetable broth

1 cup vegetable stock

1 14-ounce can black beans

1 jalapeno pepper, chopped

1/2 teaspoon sea salt

1 tbsp. apple cider vinegar

Optional:

1/2 cup crumbled corn tortilla chips

Chop onions and garlic. Chop red bell pepper. Cook and Serve

Directions:

Heat the olive oil on medium. Add the red onions and garlic to the pan and stir until softened, 3 to 5 minutes. Pour in broth, stock, salsa, jalapeno peppers, black beans, apple cider vinegar and salt. Boil over high heat. Reduce heat to low and simmer until heated through for about 5 minutes.

Vegan Chorizo and White Bean Tortilla Soup

Ingredients:

1 teaspoon extra virgin olive oil

1/2 cup chopped red onions

4 cloves garlic, minced

2 cups vegetable broth

1 cup coarsely chopped vegan chorizo

1 14-ounce can white beans

1 green bell pepper, chopped

1/2 teaspoon sea salt

1 tsp. cumin

1 tsp. paprika

1/2 cup loosely-packed cilantro

Optional:

1/2 cup crumbled corn tortilla chips

Directions:

Chop onions and garlic. Chop red bell pepper. Heat the olive oil on medium. Add the red onions and garlic to the pan and stir until softened, 3 to 5 minutes. Pour in broth, chorizo, bell peppers, cumin, black beans, paprika, and salt. Boil over high heat. Reduce heat to low and simmer until heated through for about 5 minutes.

Parsnip and Turnip Soup

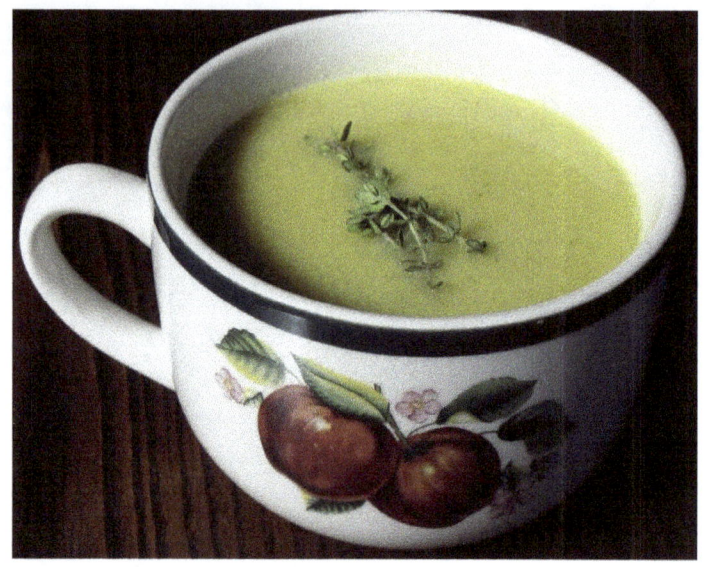

Ingredients

1 tablespoon extra-virgin olive oil

3 teaspoons crushed garlic

1 tablespoon chopped fresh cilantro

1 teaspoon chili paste

1 red onion, chopped

3 large parsnips, peeled and sliced

1 large turnip, peeled and chopped

5 cups vegetable stock

Directions:

Heat oil in a pot over medium heat. Cook garlic, cilantro and chili paste. Cook onions until tender. Add the parsnips and turnip. Cook for 5 minutes and pour in vegetable stock. Simmer for 40 minutes, or until parsnips and turnip become soft. Blend until smooth.

Jalapeno Turnip and Carrot Soup

Ingredients

1 tablespoon extra-virgin olive oil

3 teaspoons crushed garlic

1 tablespoon chopped fresh cilantro

1 teaspoon jalapeno, minced

1 tsp. cumin

1 red onion, chopped

3 large carrots, peeled and sliced

1 large turnip, peeled and chopped

5 cups vegetable stock

Directions:

Heat oil in a pot over medium heat. Cook garlic, cilantro, cumin and jalapenos. Cook onions until tender. Add the carrots and turnip. Cook for 5 minutes and pour in vegetable stock. Simmer for 40 minutes, or until turnip and carrots become soft. Blend until smooth.

Ancho Chili Carrot and Turnip Soup

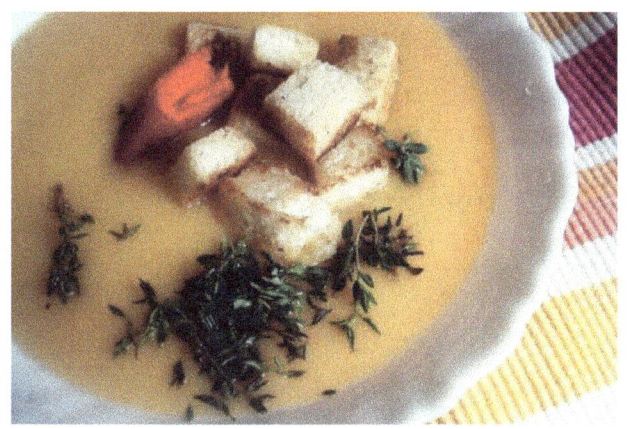

Ingredients

1 tablespoon extra-virgin olive oil

3 teaspoons crushed garlic

1 tablespoon chopped fresh cilantro

1 teaspoon lemon juice

1 teaspoon annatto seeds

½ tsp. cayenne pepper

1 teaspoon ancho chilies, finely minced

1 red onion, chopped

3 large carrots, peeled and sliced

1 large turnip, peeled and chopped

5 cups vegetable stock

Directions:

Heat oil in a pot over medium heat. Cook garlic, cilantro, lemon juice, annatto seeds, ancho chilies and cayenne pepper. Cook onions until tender. Add the carrots and turnip. Cook for 5 minutes and pour in vegetable stock. Simmer for 40 minutes, or until turnip and carrots become soft. Blend until smooth.

Hungarian Winter Squash and Carrot Soup

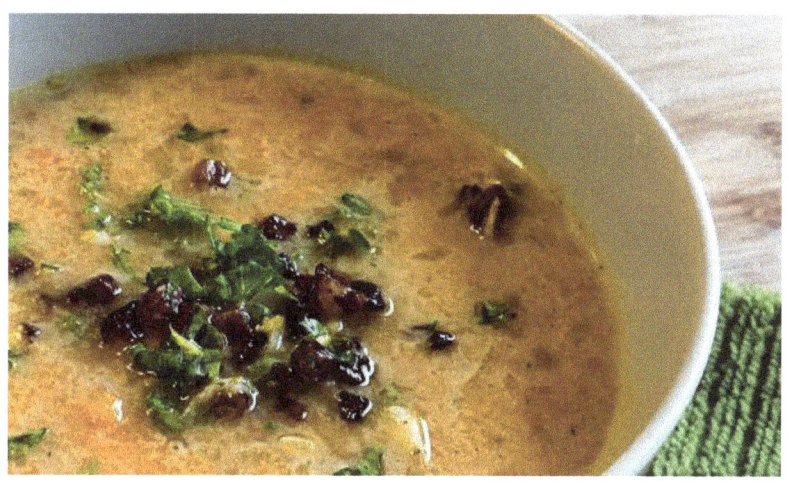

Ingredients

1 tablespoon olive oil

5 teaspoons crushed garlic

1 teaspoon Hungarian paprika

1 red onion, chopped

3 large carrots, peeled and sliced

1 large winter squash, peeled and chopped

5 cups vegetable stock

Directions:

Heat oil in a pot over medium heat. Cook garlic, cilantro and Hungarian paprika. Cook onions until tender. Add the carrots and squash. Cook for 5 minutes and pour in vegetable stock. Simmer for 40 minutes, or until winter squash and carrots become soft. Blend until smooth

Poblano Chili and Summer Squash Soup

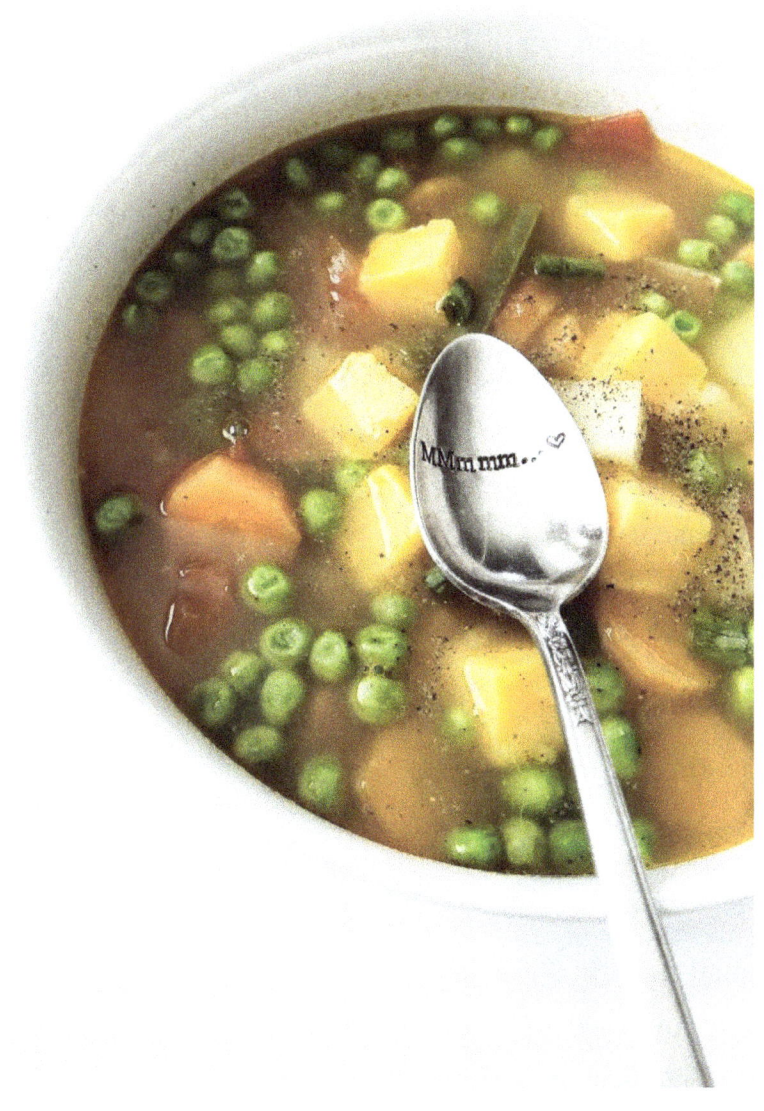

Ingredients

<u>Poblano Soup Ingredients:</u>

4 tablespoons salted butter

1 small red onion, coarsely chopped

1 large leek, white part only, sliced

1 green bell pepper, coarsely chopped

1 (or two if you like things spicy) small dry-roasted poblano chili, sliced

6 cloves garlic, diced

1 large summer squash, cubed (you can use two if you like your soup thick)

4 cups vegetable broth

1 cup cashews

1-1/4 almond milk

Sea salt

Black pepper

Directions:

Optional garnish: Sliced jalapeno pepper Soak cashews in almond milk for an hour. Melt butter in a pan. Add the red onion, leek, chilies, bell pepper, garlic, and summer squash. Cook on low heat and stir until the onion is translucent, 6 1/2 minutes. Add the broth into the pan. Simmer until the summer squash are fork tender for about 25 minutes. Take it off the heat. Process the mixture in a blender until smooth. Return the soup to the pan. In the blender, blend cashews with almond milk until smooth Add to the soup mixture. Heat the soup on medium heat for a few more minutes. Garnish with slices of jalapeno.

Creamy Potato Soup Poblano Soup

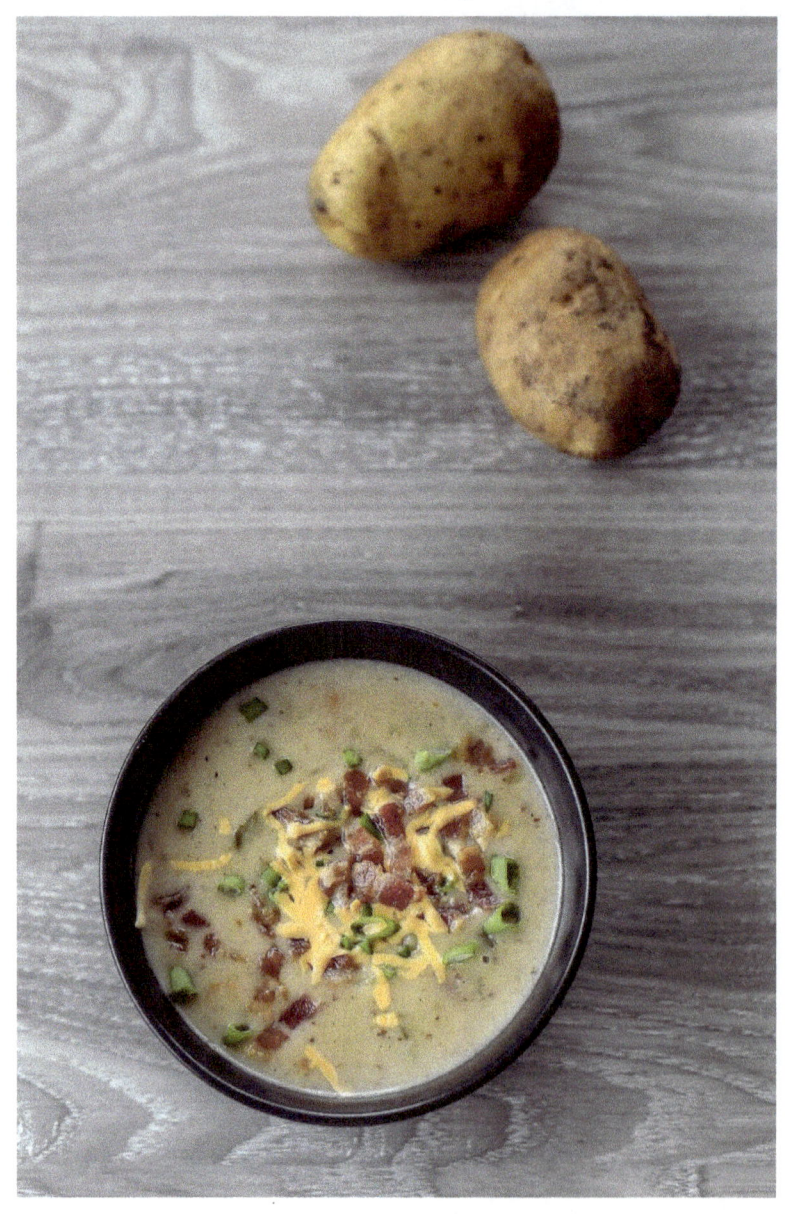

Ingredients:

4 tablespoons salted butter

1 small red onion, coarsely chopped

1 large leek, white part only, sliced

1 green bell pepper, coarsely chopped

1 (or two if you like things spicy) small dry-roasted poblano chili, sliced

6 cloves garlic, diced

1 tbsp. annatto seeds

1 large potato, cubed (you can use two if you like your soup thick)

4 cups vegetable broth

½ cup half and half

1-1/4 milk

Sea salt

Black pepper

Directions:

Optional garnish: Sliced jalapeno pepper Melt non-dairy butter in a pan. Add the red onion, leek, chilies, bell pepper, garlic, and potato. Cook on low heat and stir until the onion is translucent, 6 1/2 minutes. Add the broth and annatto seeds into the pan. Simmer until the potatoes are fork tender for about 25 minutes.

Take it off the heat. Process the mixture in a blender until smooth. Return the soup to the pan. In the blender, blend peanut butter with almond milk until smooth Add to the soup mixture. Heat the soup on medium heat for a few more minutes. Garnish with slices of jalapeno.

Borlotti Bean and Squash Soup

Ingredients

1 tablespoon extra virgin olive oil

1 small red onion, chopped

3 cloves garlic, chopped

1 tbsp. lime juice

1 cup dry borlotti beans

1 cup butternut squash - peeled, seeded, and cubed

1/3 cup finely chopped fresh cilantro

2 cups water

1/2 (14 ounce) can almond milk

2 tablespoons annatto seeds

1 teaspoon cumin

1/4 cayenne pepper

1 pinch ground nutmeg

salt and pepper to taste

Directions:

Heat the oil in a pot over medium heat Sauté the onion, garlic, annatto seeds and cumin until onion becomes tender. Add the beans, squash, and cilantro into the pot. Add the water, almond milk and lime juice Season with, cayenne pepper, nutmeg, salt, and pepper. Boil and reduce heat to low Simmer until beans and squash are tender. For about 30 min.

Spicy Summer Squash and Lentil Soup

Ingredients

1 tablespoon extra virgin olive oil

1 small red onion, chopped

3 cloves garlic, chopped

1 pinch fenugreek seeds

1 cup dry red lentils

1 cup summer squash - peeled, seeded, and cubed

1 cup water

1 cup vegetable stock

2 tablespoons tomato paste

1 teaspoon Italian seasoning

1/4 tsp. cayenne pepper

salt and pepper to taste

Directions:

Heat the oil in a pot over medium heat Sauté the onion, garlic, and fenugreek until onion becomes tender. Add the lentils and squash into the pot. Add the water, vegetable stock and tomato paste. Season with Italian seasoning, cayenne pepper, salt, and pepper. Boil and reduce heat to low Simmer until lentils and squash are tender. For about 30 min.

Chinese Turnip Soup

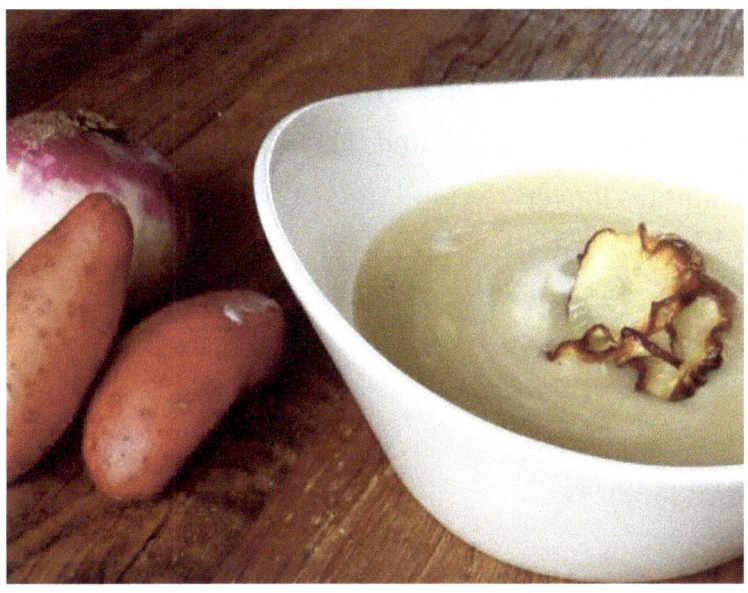

Ingredients

2 tablespoons sesame seed oil

1 small red onion, minced

1 small turnip, peeled and thinly sliced

1 celery rib, thinly sliced

1/2 teaspoon Chinese five spice powder

2 cups vegetable broth

1/4 cup rice wine

Directions:

Heat the oil over medium-high heat. Sauté red onions until tender for about 5 minutes. Slowly add turnip, celery, and five spice powder Cook for another 5 minutes, or until turnip becomes tender. Add vegetable broth and rice wine Boil and simmer. Cook for 15 minutes longer

Garnish with cilantro Spicy and Tangy Parsnip Soup

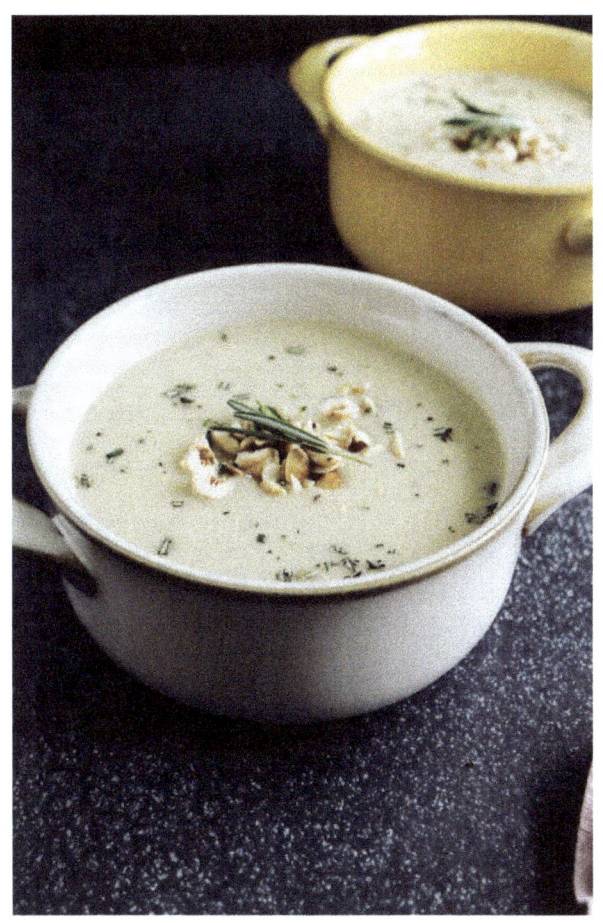

Ingredients

2 tablespoons extra virgin olive oil

1 small red onion, minced

1 small parsnip, peeled and thinly sliced

1 celery rib, thinly sliced

1/2 teaspoon cumin

½ teaspoon cayenne pepper

1 tsp. annatto seeds

1 tbsp. lime juice

2 cups vegetable stock

Directions:

Heat the oil over medium-high heat. Sauté red onions until tender for about 5 minutes. Slowly add parsnip, celery, cumin, cayenne pepper, annatto seeds and lime juice Cook for another 5 minutes, or until parsnip becomes tender. Add vegetable broth and vinegar Boil and simmer. Cook for 15 minutes longer.

Italian Vidalia Onion Soup

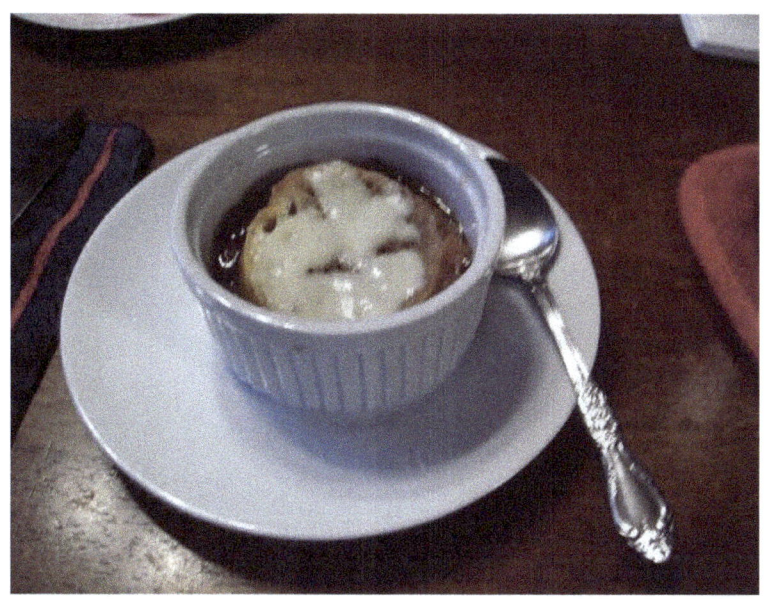

Ingredients

2 tablespoons extra virgin olive oil

2 Vidalia onions, minced

1 small carrot, peeled and thinly sliced

1 celery rib, thinly sliced

1/2 teaspoon Italian seasoning

2 cups vegetable stock

1/4 cup red wine vinegar

Directions:

Heat the oil over medium-high heat. Sauté red onions until tender for about 5 minutes. Slowly add carrots, celery, and Italian seasoning. Cook for another 5 minutes, or until carrots become tender. Add vegetable stock and red wine vinegar Boil and simmer. Cook for 15 minutes longer.

French Parsnip and Tarragon Soup

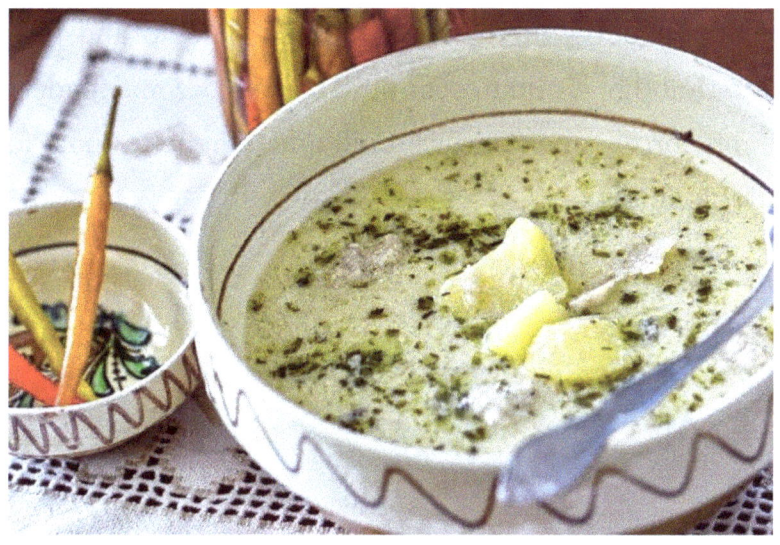

Ingredients

2 tablespoons extra virgin olive oil

1 small red onion, minced

1 large parsnip, peeled and thinly sliced

1/2 teaspoon dried tarragon

2 cups vegetable stock

1/4 cup wine vinegar

Directions:

Heat the oil over medium-high heat. Sauté red onions until tender for about 5 minutes. Slowly add parsnip and tarragon Cook for another 5 minutes, or until carrots become tender. Add vegetable broth and vinegar Boil and simmer. Cook for 15 minutes longer.

Pesto Carrot and Turnip Soup

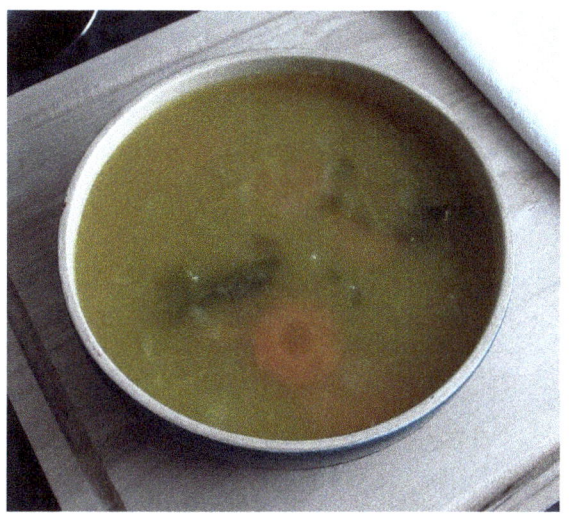

Ingredients

2 tablespoons extra virgin olive oil

1 small red onion, minced

1 medium carrot, peeled and thinly sliced

1 small turnip, peeled and thinly sliced

1/2 teaspoon dried Italian herbs

1 cup vegetable stock

1 cup vegetable broth

2 tbsp. pesto

1/4 cup wine vinegar

Directions:

Heat the oil over medium-high heat. Sauté red onions until tender for about 5 minutes. Slowly add carrots, turnip, and Italian herbs. Cook for another 5 minutes, or until carrots become tender. Add vegetable broth, stock, pesto and vinegar Boil and simmer. Cook for 15 minutes longer.

Red Onion Turnip Soup

Ingredients

2 tablespoons sesame seed oil

1 small red onion, minced

1 large turnip, peeled and thinly sliced

2 tsp. chili garlic paste

1/2 teaspoon minced ginger

2 cups vegetable broth

2 tbsp. dry sherry

2 tbsp. distilled white vinegar

1 tsp. soy sauce

Directions:

Heat the oil over medium-high heat. Sauté red onions until tender for about 5 minutes. Slowly add turnip, minced ginger, soy sauce, and chili garlic paste Cook for another 5 minutes, or until carrots become tender. Add vegetable broth, dry sherry and vinegar Boil and simmer. Cook for 15 minutes longer.

Roasted Sweet Potatoes and Green Bean Soup

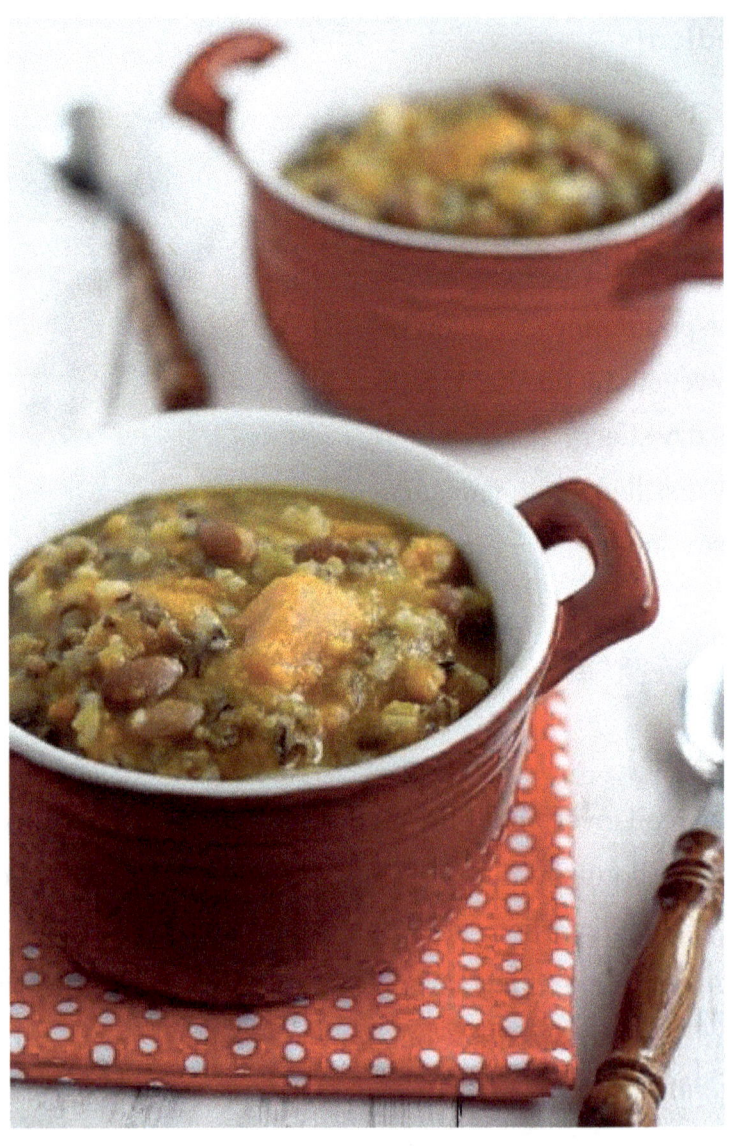

Ingredients

2 cups sweet potatoes

3 tablespoons extra virgin olive oil, divided

2 ¼ cups cherry tomatoes

2 cups

1-inch cut fresh green beans

8 cloves garlic, minced

2 teaspoons dried basil

1 teaspoon sea salt 1 (15 ounce) can lima beans, drained and rinsed

2 teaspoons extra-virgin olive oil, or to taste (optional)

Sea salt

Rainbow peppercorns to taste, finely ground

Directions:

Preheat your oven to 425 degrees F (220 degrees C). Line a baking pan with aluminum foil. Combine sweet potatoes with 1 tablespoon olive oil in a medium bowl. Pour into the baking pan. Roast in the oven until tender, for about 30 minutes. Combine the cherry tomatoes, green beans, garlic, basil, and sea salt with 2 tablespoons of olive oil. Take potatoes out of the oven Push them to one side of the pan. Add the cherry tomato and green bean mixture. Roast until the tomatoes begin to wilt, for about 18 min. Take it out of the oven and pour into a dish. Add the kidney beans, 2 teaspoons olive oil, and season with sea salt and rainbow peppercorns.

Spicy Tomato and Sweet Potato Soup

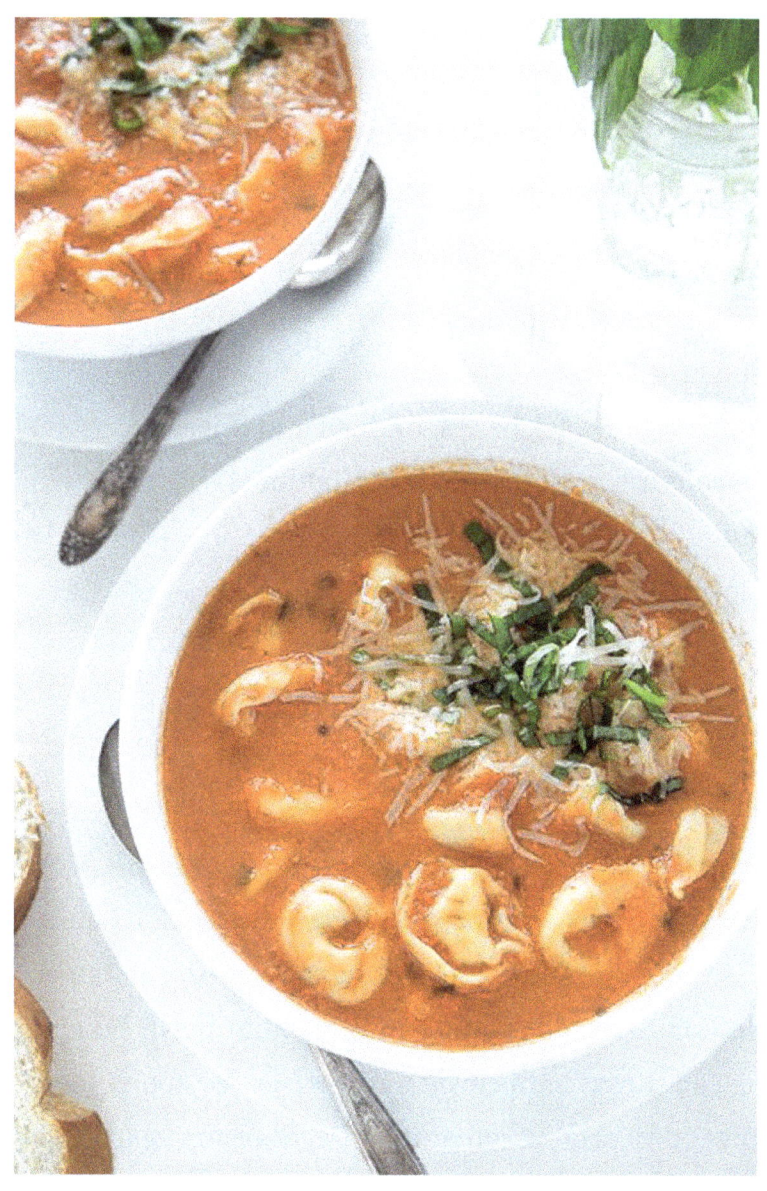

Ingredients

2 cups sweet potatoes

3 tablespoons sesame seed oil, divided

2 ¼ cups grape tomatoes

2 cups

1-inch cut fresh green beans

9 cloves garlic, minced

2 teaspoons cayenne pepper

1 teaspoon sea salt

1 (15 ounce) can black beans, drained and rinsed

2 teaspoons sesame oil, or to taste (optional)

Sea salt

Black pepper to taste

Sesame seeds for garnish

Directions:

Preheat your oven to 425 degrees F (220 degrees C). Line a baking pan with aluminum foil. Combine sweet potatoes with 1 tablespoon sesame seed oil in a medium bowl. Pour into the baking pan. Roast in the oven until tender, for about 30 minutes. Combine the cherry tomatoes, green beans, garlic, cayenne pepper, and sea salt with 2 tablespoons of sesame oil. Take potatoes out of the oven Push them to one side of the pan. Add the cherry tomato and green bean mixture. Roast until the tomatoes begin to wilt, for about 18 min. Take it out of the oven and pour into a dish. Add the black beans, 2 teaspoons sesame oil, and season with salt and pepper. Garnish with sesame seeds

Baked Smoky Broccoli and Garlic

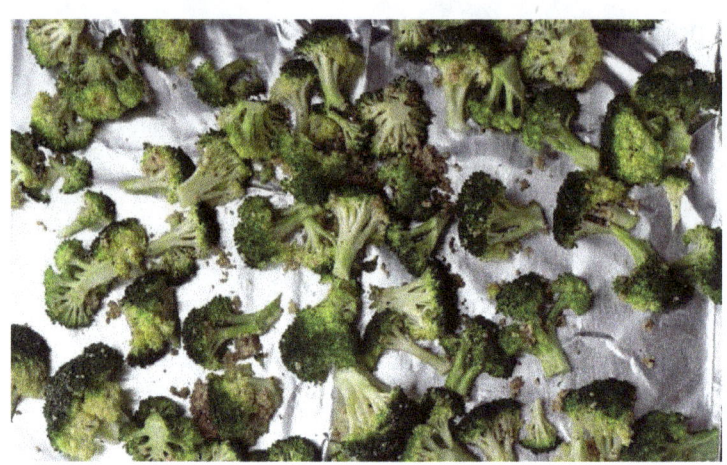

Ingredients

cooking spray

1 tablespoon extra virgin olive oil

3 cloves garlic, minced

1/2 teaspoon sea salt

1/4 teaspoon ground black pepper

½ tsp. cumin

½ tsp. annatto seeds

3 1/2 cups sliced broccoli

1 lime, cut into wedges

1 tablespoon chopped fresh cilantro

Directions:

Preheat your oven to 450 degrees F. Line a baking sheet with foil and grease with olive oil. Mix the olive oil, garlic, cumin, annatto seeds, salt, and pepper in a bowl. Add in the cauliflower, carrots, and broccoli Combine until well coated. Spread them out in a single layer on the baking sheet. Add the lime wedges. Roast in the oven until vegetables become caramelized, for about 25 minutes. Take out the lime wedges and top with the cilantro.

Asian Roasted Broccoli and Choy Sum

Ingredients

cooking spray

1 tablespoon sesame seed oil

3 cloves garlic, minced

1/2 teaspoon sea salt

1/4 teaspoon ground black pepper

3 1/2 cups sliced choy sum (Chinese Flowering Cabbage)

2 1/2 cups slice broccoli

1 tablespoon chopped fresh cilantro

Directions:

Preheat your oven to 450 degrees F. Line a baking sheet with foil and grease with olive oil. Mix the sesame oil, garlic, salt, and pepper in a bowl. Add in the choy sum and broccoli Combine until well coated. Spread them out in a single layer on the baking sheet. Roast in the oven until vegetables become caramelized, for about 25 minutes. Top with the cilantro.

Roasted Cauliflower and Lima Beans

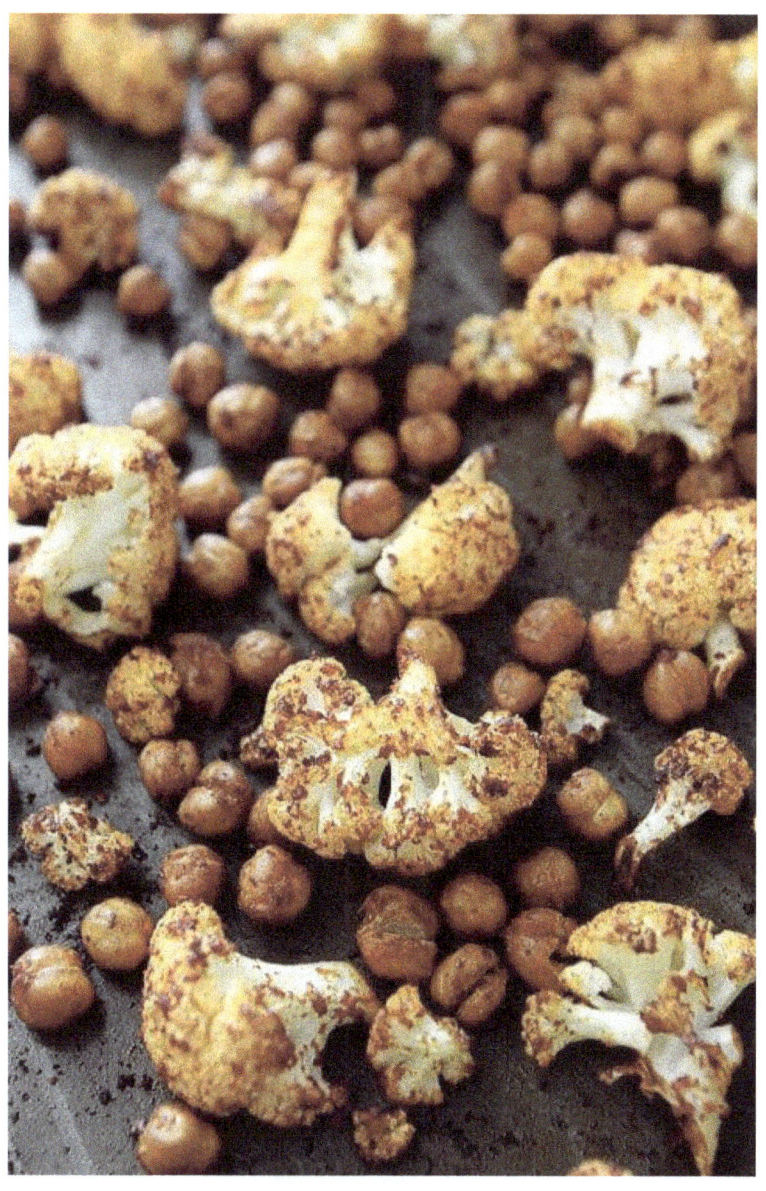

Ingredients

cooking spray

1 tablespoon melted vegan butter/margarine

9 cloves garlic, minced

1/2 teaspoon sea salt

1/4 teaspoon ground black pepper

1 1/2 cups sliced cauliflower

3 1/2 cups cherry tomatoes

1 (15 ounce) can lima beans, drained

1 lemon , cut into wedges

Directions:

Preheat your oven to 450 degrees F. Line a baking sheet with foil and grease with melted vegan butter or margarine. Mix the olive oil, garlic, salt, and pepper in a bowl. Add in the cauliflower, tomatoes, and lima beans Combine until well coated. Spread them out in a single layer on the baking sheet. Add the lemon wedges. Roast in the oven until vegetables become caramelized, for about 25 minutes. Take out the lemon wedges.

Roasted Brussel Sprouts and Choy Sum

Ingredients

cooking spray

1 tablespoon extra virgin olive oil

8 cloves garlic, minced

1/2 teaspoon sea salt

1/4 teaspoon rainbow peppercorns

3 1/2 cups sliced choy sum

2 1/2 cups sliced brussel sprouts

1 lime, cut into wedges

1 tablespoon chopped fresh cilantro

Directions:

Preheat your oven to 450 degrees F. Line a baking sheet with foil and grease with olive oil. Mix the olive oil, garlic, salt, and pepper in a bowl. Add in the choy sum and brussel sprouts Combine until well coated. Spread them out in a single layer on the baking sheet. Add the lime wedges. Roast in the oven until vegetables become caramelized, for about 25 minutes. Take out the lime wedges and top with the cilantro.

Thai Roasted Spicy Black Beans and Choy Sum

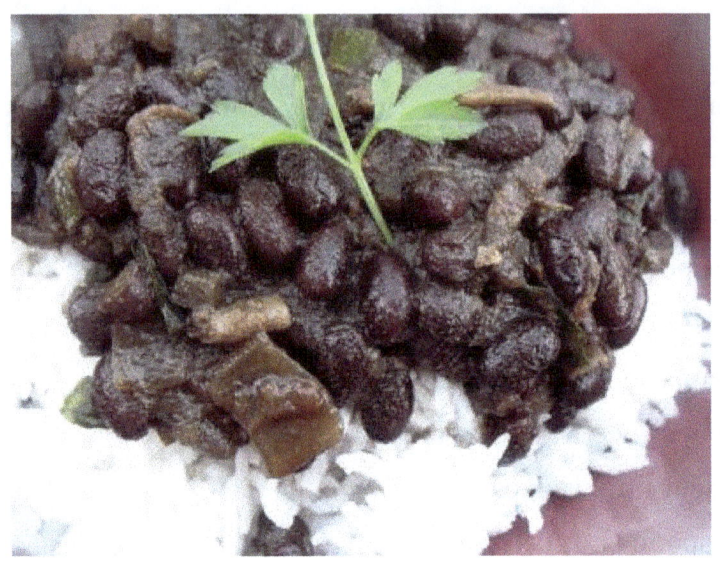

Ingredients

cooking spray

1 tablespoon sesame oil

3 cloves garlic, minced

1/2 teaspoon sea salt

1 tbsp. Thai chili paste

1/4 teaspoon ground black pepper

3 1/2 cups Choy Sum, coarsely chopped

2 1/2 cups cherry tomatoes

1 (15 ounce) can black beans, drained

1 lime, cut into wedges

1 tablespoon chopped fresh cilantro

Directions:

Preheat your oven to 450 degrees F. Line a baking sheet with foil and grease with sesame oil. Mix the olive oil, garlic, salt, Thai chili paste, and pepper in a bowl. Add in the choy sum, tomatoes, and black beans Combine until well coated. Spread them out in a single layer on the baking sheet. Add the lime wedges. Roast in the oven until vegetables become caramelized, for about 25 minutes. Take out the lime wedges and top with the cilantro.

Simple Roasted Broccoli and Cauliflower

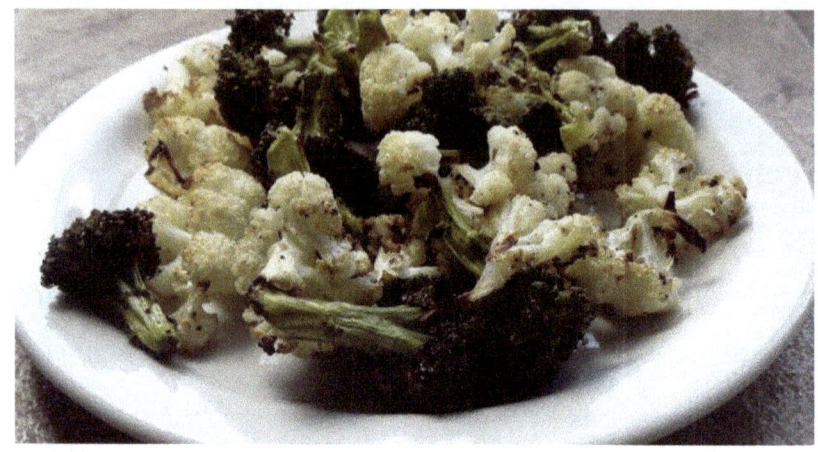

Ingredients

cooking spray

1 tablespoon extra virgin olive oil

3 cloves garlic, minced

1/2 teaspoon sea salt

1/4 teaspoon ground black pepper

3 1/2 cups broccoli florets

2 1/2 cups cauliflower florets

1 tablespoon chopped fresh thyme

Directions:

Preheat your oven to 450 degrees F. Line a baking sheet with foil and grease with olive oil. Mix the olive oil, garlic, salt, and pepper in a bowl. Add in the cauliflower and tomatoes Combine until well coated. Spread them out in a single layer on the baking sheet. Roast in the oven until vegetables become caramelized, for about 25 minutes. Top with the thyme. Simple

Roasted Spinach and Mustard Greens Extra

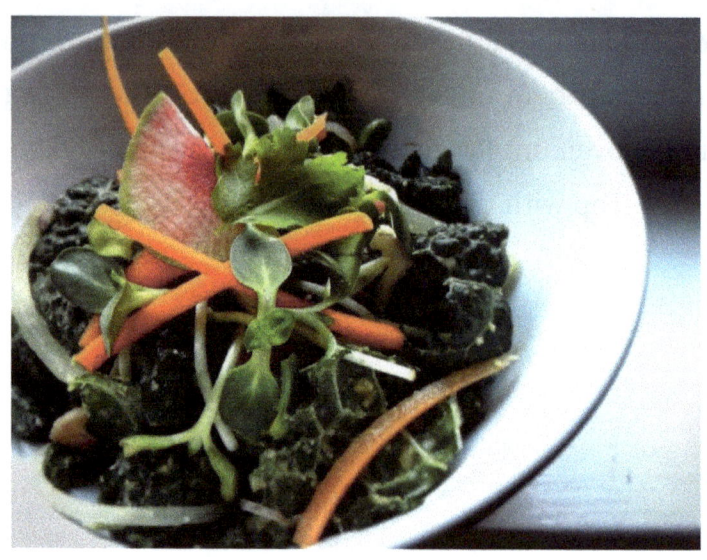

Ingredients

cooking spray

1 tablespoon extra virgin olive oil

1/2 teaspoon sea salt

1/4 teaspoon ground black pepper

Main Ingredients

1 bunch of mustard greens, rinsed and drained

1 bunch of spinach, rinsed and drained

Directions:

Preheat your oven to 450 degrees F. Line a baking sheet with foil and grease with olive oil. Mix the extra Ingredients thoroughly. Add in the main Ingredients Combine until well coated. Spread them out in a single layer on the baking sheet. Roast in the oven until vegetables become caramelized, for about 25 minutes.

Roasted Napa Cabbage and Turnips Extra

Ingredients

cooking spray

1 tablespoon extra virgin olive oil

1/2 teaspoon sea salt

1/4 teaspoon ground black pepper

<u>Main Ingredients</u>

1/2 medium Napa cabbage, sliced thinly

1 medium turnip, sliced thinly

Directions:

Preheat your oven to 450 degrees F. Line a baking sheet with foil and grease with olive oil. Mix the extra Ingredients thoroughly. Add in the main Ingredients Combine until well coated. Spread them out in a single layer on the baking sheet. Roast in the oven until vegetables become caramelized, for about 25 minutes.

Simple Roasted Kale Artichoke Heart and Choy Sum Extra

Ingredients

cooking spray

1 tablespoon extra virgin olive oil

1/2 teaspoon sea salt

1/4 teaspoon ground black pepper

Main Ingredients

1 bunch of kale, rinsed and drained

1 cup canned artichoke hearts

1/2 medium Chinese flowery cabbage (choy sum), coarsely chopped

Directions:

Preheat your oven to 450 degrees F. Line a baking sheet with foil and grease with olive oil. Mix the extra Ingredients thoroughly. Add in the main Ingredients Combine until well coated. Spread them out in a single layer on the baking sheet. Roast in the oven until vegetables become caramelized, for about 25 minutes.

Chinese Roasted Button Mushrooms and Butternut Squash

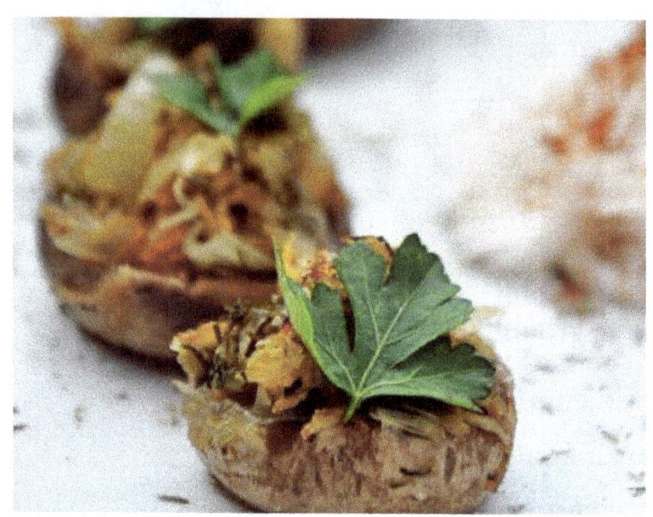

Ingredients

2 (15 ounce) cans button mushrooms, sliced and drained

1/2 butternut squash - peeled, seeded, and cut into 1-inch pieces

1 red onion, diced

2 large carrots, cut into

1 inch pieces

3 medium turnips, cut into 1-inch pieces

3 tablespoons sesame oil

Seasoning ingredients

1 teaspoon salt

1/2 teaspoon ground black pepper

1 teaspoon onion powder

2 teaspoon garlic powder

1 teaspoon Sichuan peppercorns

1 teaspoon Chinese five-spice powder

<u>Garnishing Ingredients</u>

2 green onions, chopped (optional)

Directions:

Preheat your oven to 350 degrees F. Grease your baking pan. Combine the main ingredients on the prepared sheet pan. Drizzle with the oil and toss to coat. Combine the seasoning ingredients in a bowl Sprinkle them over the vegetables on the pan and toss to coat with seasonings. Bake in the oven for 25 minutes. Stir frequently until vegetables are soft and lightly browned and chickpeas are crisp, for about 20 to 25 minutes more. Season with more salt and black pepper to taste, top with the green onion before serving.

Roasted Kale and Bok Choy Extra

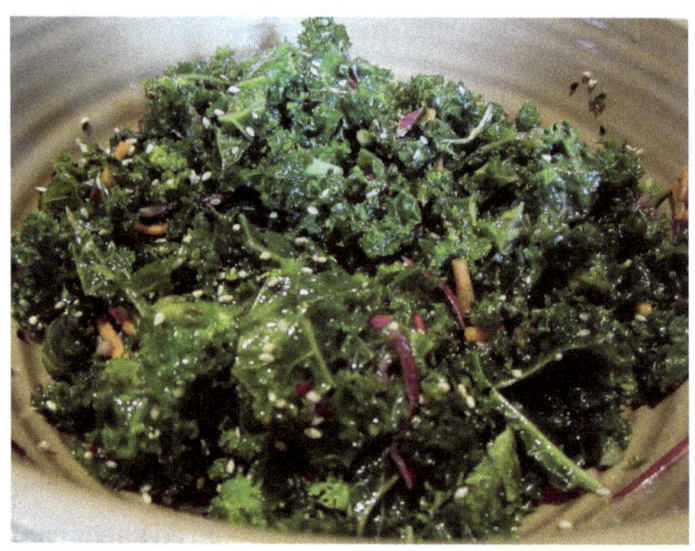

Ingredients

cooking spray

1 tablespoon extra virgin olive oil

1/2 teaspoon sea salt

1/4 teaspoon ground black pepper

Main Ingredients

1 bunch of kale, rinsed and drained

1 bunch of bok choy, rinsed, drained and coarsely chopped

Directions:

Preheat your oven to 450 degrees F. Line a baking sheet with foil and grease with olive oil. Mix the extra Ingredients thoroughly. Add in the main Ingredients Combine until well coated. Spread them out in a single layer on the baking sheet. Roast in the oven until vegetables become caramelized, for about 25 minutes.

Roasted Lima Beans and Summer Squash

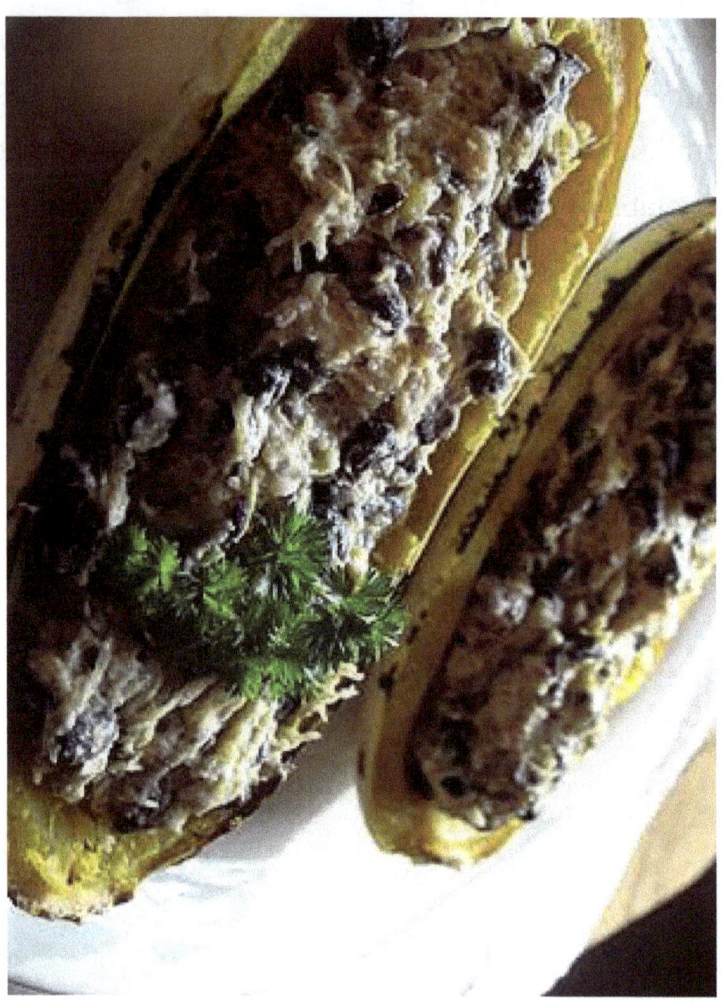

Ingredients

2 (15 ounce) cans lima beans, rinsed and drained

1/2 summer squash - peeled, seeded, and cut into

1-inch pieces

1 red onion, diced

1 sweet potato, peeled and cut into 1-inch cubes

2 large carrots, cut into 1 inch pieces

3 medium potatoes, cut into 1-inch pieces

3 tablespoons sesame oil

<u>Seasoning Ingredients</u>

1 teaspoon salt

1/2 teaspoon ground black pepper

1 teaspoon onion powder

2 teaspoon garlic powder

1 teaspoon ground fennel seeds

1 teaspoon dried rubbed sage

<u>Garnishing Ingredients</u>

2 green onions, chopped (optional)

Directions:

Preheat your oven to 350 degrees F. Grease your baking pan. Combine the beans, summer squash, onion, sweet potato, carrots, and russet potatoes on the prepared sheet pan. Drizzle with the oil and toss to coat. Combine the seasoning Ingredients in a bowl Sprinkle them over the vegetables on the pan and toss to coat with seasonings. Bake in the oven for 25 minutes. Stir frequently until vegetables are soft and lightly browned and beans are crisp, for about 20 to 25 minutes more. Season with more salt and black pepper to taste, top with the green onion before serving.

Roasted Soy Beans and Winter Squash

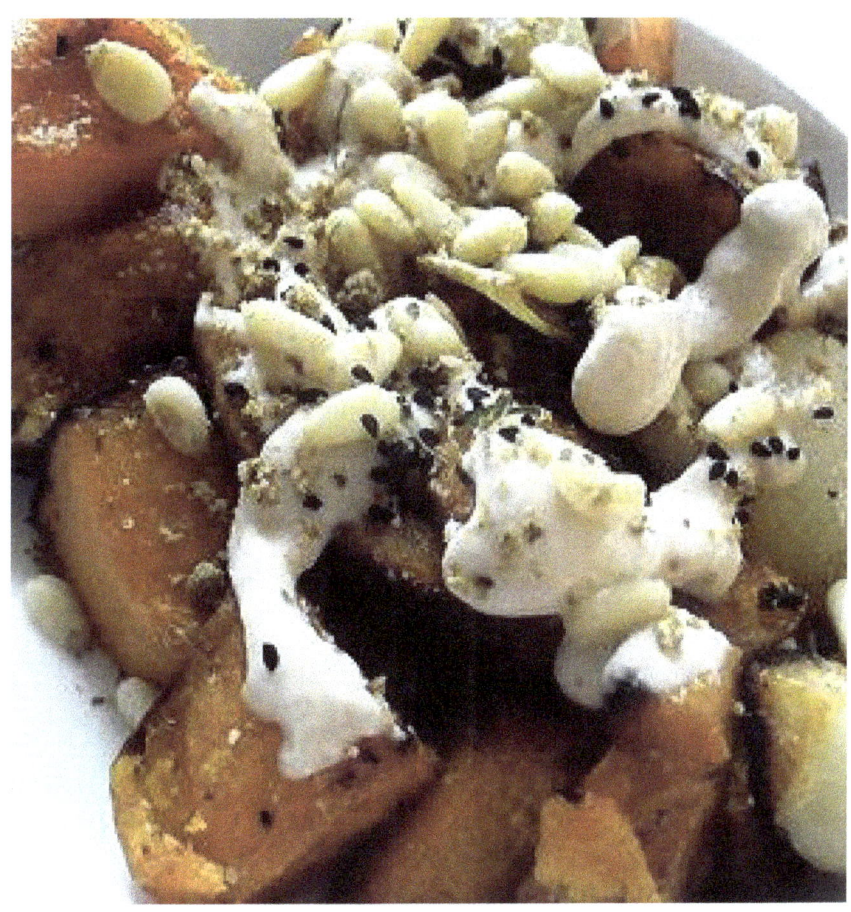

Ingredients

2 (15 ounce) cans soy beans, rinsed and drained

1/2 winter squash - peeled, seeded, and cut into 1-inch pieces

1 red onion, diced

1 sweet potato, peeled and cut into 1-inch cubes

2 large carrots, cut into 1 inch pieces

3 medium potatoes, cut into 1-inch pieces

4 tablespoons extra virgin oil

Seasoning Ingredients

1 teaspoon salt

1/2 teaspoon ground black pepper

1 teaspoon onion powder

1 teaspoon dried basil

1 teaspoon Italian seasoning

Garnishing Ingredients

2 green onions, chopped (optional)

Directions:

Preheat your oven to 350 degrees F. Grease your baking pan. Combine the beans, squash, onion, sweet potato, carrots, and russet potatoes on the prepared sheet pan. Drizzle with the oil and toss to coat. Combine the seasoning Ingredients in a bowl Sprinkle them over the vegetables on the pan and toss to coat with seasonings. Bake in the oven for 25 minutes. Stir frequently until vegetables are soft and lightly browned and beans are crisp, for about 20 to 25 minutes more. Season with more salt and black pepper to taste, top with the green onion before serving.

www.ingramcontent.com/pod-product-compliance
Lightning Source LLC
Chambersburg PA
CBHW070734030426
42336CB00013B/1969